Researching Racism in Nursing

I0131755

Research shows that racism affects the working lives of nurses and nurse academics, as well as health care service delivery and outcomes. This book looks at the impact of racism, from experiences of microaggression to discrimination and structural and institutionalised racism.

Focusing on the work of six doctoral researchers and practitioners who have chosen to address and investigate the racism they experience, witness or observe in the UK's National Health Service and Universities, this book includes personal reflections on their findings. The substantive chapters are framed by a discussion of policy and research on racism, thoughts on research supervision within this field and a drawing together of the key themes developed through this book.

Giving voice to nurses' and lecturers' responses to racism in nursing education and practice, this is an important contribution for students, researchers and practitioners with an interest in health inequalities, health care organisations, research methods and workforce development.

Helen Allan is Professor in Nursing at Middlesex University, UK.

Michael Traynor is Professor of Nursing Policy at Middlesex University, UK.

Routledge Research in Nursing and Midwifery

Birthing Outside the System
The Canary in the Coal Mine
Edited by Hannah Dahlen, Bashi Kumar-Hazard and Virginia Schmied

Nursing and Humanities
Graham McCaffrey

Grading Student Midwives' Practice
A Case Study Exploring Relationships, Identity and Authority
Sam Chenery-Morris

Complexity and Values in Nurse Education
Dialogues on Professional Education
Edited by Martin Lipscomb

Nursing Theory, Postmodernism, Post-structuralism, and Foucault
Olga Petrovskaya

Substance Use, End of Life Care and Multiple Deprivation
Practice and Research
Edited by Gary Witham, Sarah Galvani, Sam Wright and Gemma A. Yarwood

Nursing a Radical Imagination
Moving from Theory and History to Action and Alternate Futures
Edited by Jess Dillard-Wright, Jane Hopkins-Walsh, and Brandon Brown

Researching Racism in Nursing
Reflexive Accounts and Personal Stories
Edited by Helen Allan and Michael Traynor

For more information about this series, please visit:
https://www.routledge.com/Routledge-Research-in-Nursing/book-series/RRIN

Researching Racism in Nursing
Reflexive Accounts and Personal Stories

Edited by
Helen Allan and Michael Traynor

Routledge
Taylor & Francis Group

LONDON AND NEW YORK

Designed cover image: Routledge

First published 2024
by Routledge
4 Park Square, Milton Park, Abingdon, Oxon OX14 4RN

and by Routledge
605 Third Avenue, New York, NY 10158

Routledge is an imprint of the Taylor & Francis Group, an informa business

British Library Cataloguing-in-Publication Data
A catalogue record for this book is available from the British Library

ISBN: 978-1-032-21763-5 (hbk)
ISBN: 978-1-032-61526-4 (pbk)
ISBN: 978-1-003-26991-5 (ebk)

DOI: 10.4324/9781003269915

Typeset in Sabon
by codeMantra

Contents

Acknowledgements

We would like to thank colleagues over the years in the Department of Nursing and Midwifery, Middlesex University, for their engagement with ideas around racism, race and ethnicity in Nursing and Midwifery. These have been the subject of departmental seminars over some years. Many of these conversations have been translated into the doctoral work contained in this book.

Contributors

Helen Allan is Professor of Nursing at Middlesex University. Her first research study into overseas nurses' experience of working in the UK was in the mid-2000s with the Royal College of Nursing. This was published in 2003 as 'We Need Respect'. From that followed her second which was a large qualitative project exploring career progression of overseas nurses working in the UK in the mid-late 2000s, published as 'Valuing and Recognising the Talents of a Diverse Healthcare Workforce' in 2008. She has subsequently written several articles in the field and supervised PhDs exploring the experiences of overseas migrant nurses in the UK.

Dr Petula Gordon is a clinical nurse specialist. She works as an independent contractor, specialising in Infection Prevention and Control. Passionate about the mental, physical and social well-being of nurses, her research study explored the experiences of Black nurses when applying to access training and development programmes. Petula also has a keen interest in 'Clinical Supervision,' a forum that provides a safe space where nurses can reflect on their practice and explore their own personal and emotional reactions to their work.

Dr Helena Ann Mitchell has contributed extensively to mental health nursing practice and nurse education in designing, managing and leading undergraduate courses and postgraduate modules. She came to England from Guyana in 1976 to train as a registered nurse. She progressed to become a specialist community mental health nurse and then a pre-registration and post qualification lead in nurse education. She was awarded a PhD from the University of Surrey in 2015 for her study, using participatory action research, with Guyanese women living with Type 2 diabetes in England. Funding from the British Academy enabled her, as Principal Investigator, to conduct an interdisciplinary community mental health resilience project in Guyana. This commenced in February 2019 and completed in November 2020.

In January 2021 Helena Ann joined the RCN Mental Health Forum Committee, helping to shape the RCN's response to the government's consultation on reforming the Mental Health Act. She believed the mental health issues facing ethnic minority groups had not been addressed. This led to the launch of the RCN ethnic minority subgroup. Setting up this subgroup has provided the space for like-minded ethnic minority individuals to come together to address the inequality and health outcomes and generate change.

Gabriel Ngalomba was born and raised in Tanzania and moved to the UK in the 1990s. As a health care professional, he developed a passion for supporting women with perinatal mental illness to get well and return home with their babies. His particular interest has been in the Sub-Saharan African migrant women because of his heritage. This motivated him to conduct research involving this group of migrant women who experience what appeared to be racism at institutional and individual levels. Through various platforms such as this research as summarised in his chapter on racism, he believes it is possible to eradicate the racial trauma experienced by people of colour.

He remembers the saying 'Once one sees a problem s/he has to speak out in order to have the problem sorted'.

David Ring is a senior lecturer in nursing at Middlesex University and a former community-based palliative care clinical nurse specialist with a background in cancer nursing. He is a nursing PhD candidate writing a thesis titled 'An Ethnographic Study of the Experiences of Muslims Studying Nursing in London'.

David is interested in antiracism in nursing, particularly Islamophobia. David is using the products of his PhD research to develop roles in talking to white people about racism, our privilege and how we can take responsibility and work towards creating a more just system.

Donna Marie Scholefield is a senior nursing lecturer at Middlesex University, and has a background in biological science and a keen interest in pharmacological nursing. She is a co-editor of two editions of *Pharmacology Case Studies for Nurse Prescribers*. In her clinical work, she specialised in cardiac nursing, serving in different settings such as coronary care in the UK and neonatal cardiac intensive care in Riyadh, Saudi Arabia. Donna is currently pursuing a PhD and working on a thesis that explores the experience of ethnic minority academics in higher education in the UK. She has previously co-authored a publication on the implications of racism on nursing education.

Dr Iyore Monday Ugiagbe is a registered nurse, lecturer, practice educator and researcher. Ugiagbe has a clinical nursing background and senior management positions in UK national health care (NHS). He is a senior nurse lecturer and Pre-registration Adult Nursing Programme Leader at a London University. He is a listed member of the Department of Health steering group on the supervised practice programme committee that produced the first supervised practice programme for training overseas nurses during their adaptation programme to gain the UK Nursing and Midwifery Council (NMC) registration. His work revolves mainly around equality, diversity and inclusivity issues in nurse education, policy formulation and practice. He has a keen research interest in nurse education, educational measurement and evaluation, integrating internationally educated nurses in UK health care and focusing on internationally educated nurses' experiences working in the UK. Dr Ugiagbe is a certified Myers Briggs Type Indicator (MBTI) assessor and competent Thomas Kilmann Indicator (TKI) user in conflict resolution and offers support to clinical areas to resolve conflicts and to ensure a suitable/adequate clinical learning environment for the pre-registration nurses and clinical staff.

Michael Traynor was born in London. He read English Literature at Cambridge University, then completed nursing and health visiting training. He moved to Australia, where he was a researcher for the South Australian Health Commission. He worked at the Royal College of Nursing in London and at the Centre for Policy in Nursing Research at the London School of Hygiene & Tropical Medicine. He was until recently Professor of Nursing Policy at the Centre for Critical Research in Nursing and Midwifery at Middlesex University and is now an independent scholar and writer about UK nursing. He is Editor of the journal *Health*: an interdisciplinary journal for the social study of health, illness and medicine. He wrote *Critical Resilience for Nurses*, published by Routledge in March 2017, and *Stories of Resilience in Nursing*, 2020.

Foreword

I am delighted to contribute a Foreword to this book, *Researching Racism in Nursing*, which comprehensively examines the political, societal and occupational experiences of racism against the Global Ethnic Majority nursing and midwifery workforce and patient groups in the UK. This work highlights the importance of nurses taking a stand against institutional, systemic and systematic racism through the creation of doctoral research. The terminology used in this book is Black Asian Ethnic Majority (BAME) or Black Minority Ethnic (BME) in some of the research chapters.

The COVID-19 pandemic has underscored the disproportionate number of frontline health care worker deaths, while George Floyd's death in May 2020 has brought to light the overwhelming evidence of continuing racial inequality. This book is timely amid cultural and organisational changes in British nursing institutions (the Nursing Midwifery Council, NHS England and the Royal College of Nursing [RCN]).

As of 2023, since I became President of the RCN, I am a proud witness of events and steps taken in tackling racism. The Carr Review of 2022 highlighted the need for organisational and cultural change in the RCN, especially considering that 44% of its members are Global Ethnic Majority. Michelle Cox's landmark case (supported by the RCN) against NHS England/NHS Improvement was proven racism. At the Brighton Congress in 2023, the Mary Seacole Lecture took front and centre stage with Dame Elizabeth Anionwu and Professor Carole Baxter, marking a milestone for the RCN. Moreover, in my first opening speech at the congress, I included the term 'anti-racism'. This was the first time for an RCN President. RCN members voted to transform the RCN into an anti-racist organisation, a decision that would have been unheard of five years ago.

As a junior nursing academic, I began my nursing career at Middlesex University in 2014. I had faced numerous instances of racism in my career and was determined to demonstrate my worth when co-leading the Transition to Nursing Module for overseas educated nurses and changing their experiences as they were introduced to British nursing and life in the UK. During my postgraduate certificate in Higher Education (PGcert HE) at Middlesex University, I encountered Professor Helen Allan. In my write-ups, I referred to Professor Allan's publications, which provided valuable insights into the issue of racism. This association continued as I pursued my master's degree in Higher Education, where I had the good fortune to work alongside many of the authors of this book. They helped me improve my nursing teaching skills through their expert guidance. Their leadership, inspirational encouragement and influence have significantly impacted me as the then-future RCN President. Professor Allan was recently awarded an RCN Fellowship at the Brighton 2023 Congress in recognition of her research into the experiences of overseas educated nurses. Professor Michael Traynor is also a valued RCN fellow.

With these colleagues' support and guidance, I led The Healthcare Academic's Race Equality Diversity and Inclusivity Networks and the Middlesex Anti-Racism Network. These networks were initially focused on nurses, student nurses and newly qualified nurses and have been instrumental in developing and building support. I am eternally grateful to Donna Scholefield, David Ring, Sarah Chitongo and Dr Iyore Monday Ugiagbe for their unwavering encouragement, support and leadership. Their efforts have profoundly impacted me in bringing about change at the heart of the RCN in my current role as President.

The authors of this book are not only experienced nursing and midwifery clinicians but also researchers. Through their diverse and personal perspectives on critical race theory, intersectionality and other theories and philosophies, they shed light on how racism affects the mental health and well-being of patients, student nurses, registered nurses and midwives, both personally and professionally in the workplace. The writers of this book have improved people's lives as nurses and midwives. This book will be an invaluable resource for those who wish to become advocates against racism through health care and nursing research, as well as authentic allies.

Citing Professor Calvin Moorley, I 'unapologetically' connect to this book my experiences of being an Asian 'other' with a mixed religious background as a student nurse, registered nurse and academic nurse. Nurses like me have witnessed and experienced first-hand racism directed overtly and covertly towards themselves, patients, students, nurses and midwives in clinical and workplace settings.

This book is a crucial tool in the fight against institutionalised racism and the harmful anti-woke ideology that denies the existence of racism in health care. It challenges the belief that the Global Ethnic Majority (GEM), nurses, midwives and patients are disposable. It encourages readers to consider the impact of racism on those affected in the UK, the NHS, and on nursing shortages.

Racism is evidenced by the death of Amine Abdullah who took his own life in 2016 after being unfairly dismissed from his NHS job, and recently the

RCN Foundation has opened a grant funding opportunity in his name. The question is posed: is losing another valuable member of the nursing workforce worth it?

If the answer is no, what actions will you take to support the cause? I recommend reading the chapters of this book to begin with!

S. Sobrany
Sheilabye Sobrany (Sheila) She/Her
President of the Royal College of Nursing
RGN PGcert HE, MA HE, FEHEA

1 Introduction

Researching racism in nursing

Helen Allan

Language style

We agree with Flanigan et al.'s (2021) advice for health care researchers in their 2021 paper, Updated Guidance on the Reporting of Race and Ethnicity in Medical and Science Journals, that race and ethnicity are social constructs, without scientific or biological meaning. They do, however, have political meaning (UK Government, 2021; Rollock, 2022). While these terms have been taken to have scientific validity, concerns about the use of these terms in health care education, practice and research are now recognised (Flanigan et al., 2021). As a group of authors, we have discussed which language would best address white privilege when referring to people from black, brown, Asian or white heritage. All acronyms when referring to people's colour, race and ethnicity are reductive, inaccurate and unrepresentative of smaller groups; they imply a hierarchy between groups and eliminate differences between and within groups. Each author, therefore, uses language they believe acknowledges this. In this chapter I have used the British (albeit, itself contested) practice for referring to BAME when speaking or writing about people of colour (Brathwaite, 2018). That is, Black, Asian and minority ethnic (BAME) to refer to nurses of non-European heritage and white to refer to nurses of European heritage. BIPOC (Black, Indigenous and people of colour) may be more familiar to a North American audience, and we are mindful of the international audience who may have different views.

Seeking to understand racism

As white researcher(s) we have come to understand that racism is structurally, institutionally and culturally systemic in British society (Allan, 2021). It manifests itself directly and indirectly both at the institutional level and through interpersonal relationships (Larsen et al., 2005; Smith et al., 2008). Intentionally and unintentionally is another way of describing these interpersonal racist acts. It is a system of discrimination, oppression and white privilege (DiAngelo, 2018; Iheduru-Anderson et al., 2021) which is painfully obvious to people of colour in everyday acts of microaggressions and

DOI: 10.4324/9781003269915-1

systemic injustices (Akala, 2019) but goes unrecognised by white people who benefit from their white, racialised identities and positioning (Olusoga, 2016; DiAngelo, 2018). As such, racism is culturally as well as structurally and institutionally reproduced; that is, ideas, beliefs and values about non-white people are reproduced in cultural forms which sustain structural and institutional forms of racism. Racism is not solely caused by individual actions, beliefs or attitudes although these underpin and therefore interact with institutional policies and practices (Olusoga, 2016; Akala, 2019). Drevdahl et al. (2006) and van Herk et al. (2011) have argued that in nursing, it is commonly believed that nursing as a profession isn't racist, that racist acts are caused by individuals rather than the profession as a whole. There are some emerging studies which challenge this (Mitchell et al., 2017; Thorne, 2020). We dispute any claim that nursing isn't systemic and institutional. Our edited book goes some way to addressing this lack of research evidence of the presence of racism in nursing. Racism is built into social structures, including the structures of the nursing and midwifery professions, and as a result, is often invisible to white people (Akala, 2019) as whiteness itself is historically invisible (Olusoga, 2016; DiAngelo, 2018).

Historical overview of race and racism

In the United Kingdom (UK), the Race Relations Act (1968) outlawed discrimination on the grounds of colour, nationality and ethnic or national origins. However, while race remains a protected characteristic under The Equality Act (2010), ethnic inequalities in the education, work, health and criminal justice systems remain (Equality and Human Rights Commission, 2016). Prejudice on the basis of race is the most common form of discrimination in Europe (European Union, 2015), while in the UK, racial discrimination has increased following the national referendum to leave the European Union in 2016 (Kelley et al., 2017; Reynolds, 2019). It also has an impact on NHS service delivery and outcomes (particularly mental health outcomes although physical health as well) across the lifespan (Hackett et al., 2020), notably maternity outcomes (Knight et al., 2020). Research and personal accounts show that racism also affects the working lives of nurses and those employed as nurse lecturers in the UK (Thurman et al., 2019; Kline, 2020; Moorley et al., 2020; Cox et al., 2021).

Racism includes experiences of microaggression (Williams et al., 2020), discrimination from structural and institutionalised racism in terms of promotions and access to other social, political and economic opportunities (Smith et al., 2008; Moorley et al., 2020). At both the structural[1] and individual levels in society, racial discrimination is thought to effect health in numerous ways. At the structural level, racial discrimination may operate through the unfair allocation of societal resources that are determinants of health (e.g. education, employment, housing) and through differential access to health care, as well as poorer quality of care. Racial discrimination may also affect health through stress-related biological processes. Frequent exposure to racial discrimination is a chronic stressor and has been linked with dysregulated cardiovascular, neuroendocrine and inflammatory processes which in turn affects both physical and mental health. The social determinants of health, including ethnicity and racism, are known to cause poorer health outcomes in BAME groups and communities in the United Kingdom. The COVID pandemic has made this abundantly clear (Pan et al., 2020; Public Health England, 2020). However, the reluctance and failure of repeated governments to tackle the social determinants of health is partially explained by recognising the power of cultural racism which either ignores such differences or attributes poorer health outcomes in BAME groups and communities to cycles of deprivation which are portrayed as intractable as they care caused by cultural difference of BAME groups within British society (Marmot et al., 2020). This form of cultural racism is reproduced through the media.

The history of race and racism is an extensive one which is studied within many disciplines (legal studies, geography, feminism among others). In this introduction to race and racism, we draw on work within history and sociology which argues that current systems of racism have their origins in the history of British mercantile expansion, colonialism and Empire (Historic England, 2022):

> *Imperial European powers found ways to justify the barbaric slave system and the invasion, colonisation and expropriation of foreign lands for the expansion of their wealth. Britain amongst them created a hierarchy with white Europeans at the top and Africans and Asians at the bottom. Racism became embedded into the nation's structures of power, culture, education and identity.*
>
> (https://historicengland.org.uk/research/inclusive-heritage/another-england/a-brief-history/racism-and-resistance/.
> Accessed: January 2022)

Olusoga (2016) argues that racism needs to be understood in the context of discourses about race which have for several centuries provided the basis for relationships between black and non-white people. These discourses have emphasised the differences between people based on skin colour. In his book *Black and British, A Forgotten History*, he argues that medieval beliefs that black skin was a marker for servitude was a justification for the slave trade, colonialism and the building of Empires by European powers from the 16th century onwards. As Kendi (2020) argues, racists have always accentuated differences between groups that don't exist and ignored differences (inequalities, bias, discrimination) that do. And current systems of institutional and structural racism where BAME ethnic groups are systemically at a racial disadvantage in the UK (and elsewhere) is based on the legacies of the British slave trade and colonialism (Olusoga, 2016; DiAngelo, 2018). There is still reluctance among white people and society to recognise this legacy (Zack, 2002; Saini, 2019).

Racist systems give rise to racist institutional practices, which are reproduced by individuals in everyday life, and are based on a relationships between BAME and white people which became to be seen as the 'natural order of society' in Britain (Olusoga, 2016). However, to understand racism we need to understand the concept of race. What is the meaning of race? To answer this we need to briefly discuss so-called 'scientific' theories of race (Skibba, 2019).

Theories of race

Olusoga (2016) argues that with mercantile expansionism and the early British trading Empire in the 15th and16th centuries, an explanation of difference in skin colour and other cultural differences developed as a biological taxonomy of races which became an early form of cultural racism. A belief in a taxonomy of races was further entrenched during the Enlightenment in the 18th century by the new scientific method which sought to explain observed differences between people in the emerging global empires (Zack, 2002). This new science of race, or scientific racism (Olusoga, 2016) built on pre-Enlightenment beliefs expressed in the taxonomy of races. These provided a blueprint for the ideologies underpinning imperialism, colonialism and slavery, racial segregation and genocide which exist today (Zack, 2002; Saini, 2019). Lippert-Rasmussen (2006) argues that scientific understanding of differences which were observed between peoples informed racialism, the belief in biologically distinct human races, as well as racism, which accorded a hierarchy of value to difference where white was seen as morally, socially, politically, religiously and economically higher than black or brown skin.

The meanings of both race and ethnicity have changed over time and continue to do so. The first usage of race was in the 1500s (Bell, 1995; Olusoga, 2016; Flanigan et al., 2021) while ethnicity was first used in the late 1700s (Olusoga, 2016). The Oxford English Dictionary (OED, 2021) defines race as 'a group of people connected by common descent or origin' or 'any of the (putative) major groupings of mankind, usually defined in terms of distinct physical features or shared ethnicity'. The Collins English Dictionary (2021) specifically mentions skin colour as a determinant of race: '*A race is one of the major groups which human beings can be divided into according to their physical features, such as the colour of their skin*'. Ethnicity is defined as '*membership of a group regarded as ultimately of common descent, or having a common national or cultural tradition*' (OED, 2021).

An example of a scientific theory of race is the much cited evidence of the differences between black and white Americans in terms of their IQ scores (Bell, 1995; Fraser, 1995). Race theory was used to explain lower intelligence (measured in IQ) in black Americans compared to white Americans (Bell, 1995). Research in the mid-late 20th century shows that the strong relationship between poorer resources (economic, political and social) predicts these lower scores rather than any biological or cognitive explanation (Bell, 1995). Hilario et al. (2017) cite Drevdahl et al. (2001, 311) who argue that '*the results of living in a racialized society very often lead to biological differences in health*'. In other words, there are differences between groups in society but these are caused by society rather than by essentialist differences between groups (Kendi, 2020). Scientific racism has had severe (literally fatal) and lasting psychological, social, economic and political consequences over generations. Bell (1995, 895) links the history of black oppression with recent outrage over the social and economic oppression of black Americans thus:

> *As history indicates all too well, blacks have suffered greatly as a result of discrimination undergirded and often justified by the general belief in black inferiority.*

Similar arguments have been made since the *#BlackLivesMatters* protests started globally (Lebron, 2017). Sociology but also society is in the middle of an 'unfinished conversation' about race and ethnicity (Solomos, 2020).

Scientific racism was based on an ideology of race (Bell, 1995; Andrews et al., 2014; Hilario et al., 2017) and it was debunked and rejected in the 20th century as the relationship between ideology and the scientific method, the practice and write-up of science, was understood in critical theory in the 1940s onwards (Zack, 2002; Dreger, 2015; Saini, 2019). As Saini (2019) observes

> *Individual variation within population groups, overlapping with other population groups, turned out to be so large that the boundaries of race made less and less sense.... The conclusion was that no "pure" races exist that are distinct from other.*

While race and ethnicity are social constructs with no scientific basis, the terms may be useful as a lens through which to study and view racism and disparities and inequities in health, health care and medical practice, education and research. The contradiction at the heart of racism studies is that race itself is now discredited but racism exists. As Flanigan et al. (2021, 622) describe it:

> *Although race and ethnicity have no biological meaning, the terms have important, albeit contested, social meanings. Neglecting to report race and ethnicity in health and medical research disregards the reality of social stratification, injustices, and inequities and implications for population health and removing race and ethnicity from research may conceal health [and other] disparities.*

The studies described in this book show that it is the recognition of the relationship between knowledge, science and everyday experiences of race which prompted these doctoral students to engage with their topic. The authors emphasise the historical and socially embedded conceptualisations of race, racialisation and ethnicity at work in health care today in Britain, most often drawing on critical race theory (CRT). They engage with the ideas of inter-sectionality which argue that racism is not the only source of social inequality and racism does not operate in isolation (Crenshaw, 1991).

Critical race theory (CRT)

CRT originated as a way to examine, uncover and disrupt processes of racism in legal studies (Bell, 1995; Bryder, 1998). CRT is used increasingly in nursing to explore ideological, structural and institutional racism (Hilario et al., 2017; Brathwaite, 2018; Cunningham & Scarlato, 2018; Ackerman-Barger et al., 2019; Bennett et al., 2019). We understand structural racism to refer to the systematic exploitation of ethnic minority communities, which leads to material disadvantage; institutional racism refers to racism in institutional settings, political or social forces or influences, which reproduce racism through policies and practice, unconsciously or consciously. CRT illuminates the existence of colonial power and racism within the hierarchical and institutional structures of the NHS and nursing (Brathwaite, 2018). There are three separate strands to CRT: (i) racism is understood to be an everyday experience for people of colour, which is unacknowledged and difficult to address or eliminate. In not recognising or acknowledging racism, white people as individuals and simultaneously as part of wider society, do not recognise themselves as racist or part of a racist society (Clarke & Garner, 2010; DiAngelo, 2018); (ii) white people's failure to see themselves as racist leads to a failure to see the interests that they accrue as white people. These interests are economic, political and psychological; (iii) CRT views race as a social construct with no basis in biology; individuals are defined in racial terms depending on the economic and material interests of those in power (DiAngelo, 2018).

Whiteness, white privilege and white supremacy

What is whiteness? It is generally taken to denote an absence of specificity, or an invisible non-raced identity (Nayak, 2007; Garner, 2007). However, as Garner (2009) suggests, increasingly whiteness is visible both by white communities and individuals themselves (perhaps even more so in the context of the migration debates in the UK during the 2010s) and by BAME groups. He also cites fear of whiteness as a political tool to disempower BAME communities. Garner argues that:

> *Whiteness may emerge therefore as either marked (visible) or unmarked (invisible), depending on the location of the person doing the looking.*
>
> (2009, 3)

American studies (for example, Lamont, 2000) suggest that whiteness is socially constructed through what are perceived to be widely accepted, 'normal' or 'commonsense' norms and values. In constructing and performing whiteness, 'Other' is also constructed as the antithesis of whiteness (Garner, 2009). The key consequence of whiteness is white privilege.

DiAngelo (2018) argues that racism rests on white privilege (systemic and structural advantages over people of colour) and white supremacy (the belief that white people are superior to people of colour) which blinds white people to their own colour, rendering them unaware of their whiteness and the privilege this gives them. Or as Blanchett Garneau et al. (2018) describe, this is a process where the *harms of culturalist assumptions* go unrecognised and unchallenged by the white perpetrator (DiAngelo, 2018). Whiteness is therefore about power arising solely from an individual's skin colour and the privilege that this gives them in society, including access to resources at interpersonal and structural levels, which has a generational advantage. Clarke and Garner (2010, 15) describe these advantages as

> legacies of inter-generational relative advantage. However low they are in a given socio-economic order, white people benefit from being white, and not necessarily intentionally.

To this we would add that social class privileges peculiar to British nursing (Snee and Goswami, 2020) may intersect with whiteness to construct white privilege. Social class may be a reflection of white privilege in the British context. As Snee and Goswami (2020) argue, there remain class advantages for those from professional backgrounds in British nursing; the impact of social class endures to privilege male nurses particularly strongly in career progression. They argue that nursing has a 'glass ceiling' for those female nurses not from professional backgrounds. At this stage, their analysis does not include race or ethnicity as the data they draw do not have these categories.

The 'good/bad binary' and white fragility

DiAngelo's (2018) description of the good/bad binary in white people's understanding of who is a racist and the ensuing white fragility have been important to an emerging understanding of racism, racism in nursing and white privilege. DiAngelo (2018, 71) uses the phrase '*He's not racist. He is a really nice guy*' to describe the good/bad binary which is how white people imagine racists. In nursing we could say, '*she's not a racist, she's a really good nurse*'. We imagine a racist to be someone who commits 'simple, isolated and extreme acts of prejudice' (2018, 71); we believe that only bad people can be racists. DiAngelo calls the good/bad binary '*the most successful adaptation of racism in recent history*' (2018, 71). This belief prevents white people acknowledging their colour and their white privilege in structural and institutional forms of racism.

This is behind the response, *'all lives matter'* to *#BlackLivesMatter* (Stollznow, 2021). DiAngelo (2018, 107) argues that this response comes from a position where the white person fails to see themselves in racial terms, refuses to engage further with discussions of racism and in their own minds, becomes the victim of racism. This position of white fragility is powerfully socialised in white culture (Clarke & Garner, 2010).

Many of the contributors to this book have chosen to engage with CRT.

History of racism in nursing and midwifery

While racism has been shown to be prevalent in nursing and health care settings globally (Allan et al., 2004; Allan, 2007; Smith et al., 2008; Allan et al., 2009; Hall & Fields, 2012, 2013; Kline, 2014; Blanchett Garneau et al., 2018; Brathwaite, 2018; Thurman et al., 2019; Olusanya, 2021), Iheduru-Anderson et al. (2021) argue there is little acknowledgement of institutional racist practices in nursing and little awareness of how nursing is complicit in institutionally racist health services. This is not surprising given that nursing has always been a mirror of society, constrained by its social, political and economic context. Nursing is as constrained by society's beliefs and structures around race, ethnicity, gender and social class stereotypes as any other profession or public institution (Snee & Goswami, 2020). Consequently, there is denial in nursing that racism is systemic and institutional (Drevdahl et al., 2006). Where there is acknowledgement of racism, it tends to centre around individual acts of racism or individual racist nurses rather than any awareness of different levels of racism (Flanigan et al., 2021). The literature shows that there is a need to understand how racism is reproduced across different health care settings; and the struggle against racism and discrimination in nursing and health care services is ongoing (Van Herk et al., 2011; Thorne, 2020; Iheduru-Anderson et al., 2021).

Racialising processes in nursing

The language of racism is difficult for white people as it requires us to make whiteness visible and thus, our complicity in racism (DiAngelo, 2018). To avoid this discomfort, DiAngelo argues that we use other labels (social class, nationality) to avoid naming racism. I believe that the discursive repertoires of race (Frankenberg, 1994) in nursing make this even more difficult for white nurses to acknowledge the whiteness of nursing and challenge systemic racism. Clarke and Garner (2010) use 'discursive repertoires' to describe the ways in which society uses discourse to structure racism. These are where there is evasion of direct references to 'race' with discourses involving culture, nation, class and gender. These discourses may be overt or covert. DiAngelo (2018) cites covert codes for racism which emerge in American social exchanges, such as parents' talk about neighbourhoods. A nursing example from my experience was when I was told as a student and later as a clinical teacher by nurses looking after young patients with sickle cell disease, that 'those' patients do not require analgesia because 'they don't experience pain like we do' and that 'they put a lot of the pain on'. Blanchett Garneau et al. (2018) argue that existing nursing pedagogies powerfully reproduce racism; these pedagogies are entrenched, unseen and unacknowledged (van Herk et al., 2011; Hall & Fields, 2012). Pedagogies in nurse education encompass approaches to learning which include informal, incidental and formal learning which is socially constructed through interactions and relationships between lecturers and students, students' peer relationship and between students and staff in clinical teams in health care organisations (Allan & Smith, 2010). Pedagogies shape and constrain how students are socialised during their educational programmes, including their clinical placements; they shape the curriculum, the hidden curriculum, the spaces and sites of learning (Evans et al., 2010). Nursing pedagogies reproduce racism to construct a homogeneity in nursing where whiteness is dominant, unseen and invisible and BAME nurses are seen as other (Puzan, 2003). This renders talking about racism difficult if not impossible (Holland, 2015). Iheduru-Anderson et al. (2020) argue that a culture of silence around, and a collective denial of, racism, act as racialising processes in nursing both in current nurse education and practice and in historical accounts (Stake-Doucet, 2020). BAME nurses struggle to fit in (Smith et al., 2008) because difference is excluded and whiteness continues unacknowledged and unseen.

Anti-racism

There is a rich, global literature on racism in nursing (Baxter, 1988; Kushnick, 1988; Condliffe, 2001; Likupe & Archibong, 2013). There is also a long history of activism against racism (Grumbling Appendix, 2016; Blanchett Garneau et al., 2018; Thorne, 2020). Individual nurses (McKay, 2020), nursing organisations (Kinnair, 2020) and nurse academics have spoken out in support of *#BlackLivesMatter* and advocate anti-racism action (Blanchett Garneau et al., 2018). There is evidence of strategies to tackle institutional racism and unconscious bias in nursing (Dangerfield et al., 2020; Foster, 2020; Iheduru-Anderson et al., 2021). As well as a powerful critique of nursing to address the historical legacy of colonialism and racism in nursing and nurse education (Brathwaite, 2018; Stake-Doucet, 2020; Thorne, 2020).

Book overview

This book is built around the work of six doctoral candidates who, each in different ways and focusing on different topics, have chosen to address and investigate the racism they experience, witness or observe in the NHS by means of doctoral study and, in the process of their investigations, have been profoundly changed. The main body of the book sets out the research work, methodology and findings (provisional in some cases of work in progress) by each, alongside first-hand accounts of personal realisations that their work has brought about for them. This central material is framed by discussion of policy and research on racism, reflective accounts of research supervision within this field of work and a drawing together of the themes developed in each study, by each doctoral candidate. The book and the accounts within it bear witness to the claim that 'the personal is the political'.

As editors who are white, we have thought carefully both in supervision and in deciding to start this book project, about our role in both racism in nursing (how we have both benefitted from white privilege – see Allan, 2021) and in supervision when the topic of study is racism. Our supervisions have led us to reflect upon the structural domination of whiteness as it intersects with the potential of individual critique and reflexivity. And we have at times reflected upon our own positioning as white nurse researchers while supervising BAME doctoral students who are investigating the very *basis of our privilege*. As Helen acknowledges in her paper on racialised white identities in nursing (Allan, 2021) it is an irony that we have both spent a significant amount of time as researchers investigating or supervising studies which investigate racism in the NHS while ignoring our own positioning as white researchers and our own white privilege. Helen (2021) suggests that one interpretation of our failure to understand our own position in a white supremacist society is a defence against the pain of recognising our own racism, or white fragility.

This book goes beyond 'occasional performative allyship' (Moorley et al., 2020, 2451) to give voice to BAME and white nurses' and lecturers' responses to racism in nurse education and nursing practice. It is a timely attempt to respond to 'institutional forgetfulness' (Moorley et al., 2020, 2451).

Acknowledgement

Alongside the editors of this book, the supervisory teams of the contributors also include the following colleagues: Reza Gholami (University of Birmingham); Linda Collins (South Eastern Louisiana University, USA); Herminder Kaur, Venetia Brown, Catherine Kerr and Gordon Weller from Middlesex University. All of the contributors to this book thank them for their invaluable support and advice.

Note

1 By structure we mean the recurrent patterned arrangements that influence or limit the choices and opportunities available to people. At the individual level of society individuals are considered to have the capacity for agency, to act independently and make their own choices (Giddens, 1984).

References

Ackerman-Barger, K., Boatright, D., Gonzalez-Colaso, R., Orozco, R., & Latimore, D. (2019). Seeking inclusion excellence: understanding racial microaggressions as experienced by underrepresented medical and nursing students. *Academic Medicine*, **95**, 5, 758–763. doi: 10.1097/ACM.0000000000003077

Akala. (2019). *Natives Race and Class in the Ruins of Empire*. London: Hodder & Stoughton.

Allan, H. T. (2007). The rhetoric of caring and the recruitment of overseas nurses: the social reproduction of a care gap. *Journal Clinical Nursing*, **16**, 2204–2212. https://doi.org/10.1111/j.1365-2702.2007.02095

Allan, H. T. (2021). Reflections on whiteness: racialised identities in nursing. *Nursing Inquiry*, e12467. https://doi.org/10.1111/nin.12467

Allan, H. T., & Smith, P. A. (2010). Pedagogies and methodologies for nurse education research: are they used in research and evident in practice? *Nurse Education Today*, 30, 5, 476–479.

Allan, H. T., Cowie, H., & Smith, P. A. (2009). Overseas nurses' experiences of discrimination: a case of racist bullying. *Journal of Nursing Management*, 17, 898–906. doi: 10.1177/0969733010368747

Allan, H. T., Larsen, J., Bryan, K., & Smith, P. (2004). The social reproduction of institutional racism: internationally recruited nurses' experiences of the British Health Services. *Diversity in Health and Social Care*, 1, 2, 117–126.

Andrews, K., Bassel, L., & Winter, A. (2014). The British Sociological Association race and ethnicity study group conference 'mapping the field: contemporary theories of race, racism and ethnicity. *Ethnic and Racial Studies*, 37, 10, 1862–1868. https://doi.org/10.1080/01419870.2014.931994

Baxter, C. (1988). *The Black Nurse: An Endangered Species*. Cambridge: National Extension College for Training in Health and Race.

Bell, D. A. (1995). *Who's afraid of Critical Race Theory?* David C. Baum Memorial Lectures on Civil Liberties and Civil Rights at the University of Illinois College of Law. University of Illinois Law Review 1995(4). Retrieved from: http://publish.illinois.edu/lawreview/archives/volume-1995/

Bennett, B., Hamilton, E. K., & Rochani, H. D. (2019). Exploring race in nursing: Teaching nursing students about racial inequality using the historical lens. *Online Issues in Nursing*, **24**, 2. Retrieved from: https://ojin.nursingworld.org/MainMenuCategories/ANAMarketplace/ANAPeriodicals/OJIN/TableofContents/Vol-24-2019/No2-May-2019/Articles-Previous-Topics/Exploring-Race-in-Nursing.html

Blanchett Garneau, A., Browne, A. J., & Varcoe, C. (2018). Drawing on antiracist approaches toward a critical antidiscriminatory pedagogy for nursing. *Nursing Inquiry*, 5, 1, e12211. https://doi-org.ezproxy.mdx.ac.uk/10.1111/nin.12211

Brathwaite, B. (2018). Black, Asian and minority ethnic nurses: colonialism, power and racism. *British Journal of Nursing*, 27, 5, 254–258. doi: 10.12968/bjon.2018.27.5.254

Bryder, L. (1998). Sex, race, and colonialism: an historiographical review. *The International History Review*, 20, 4, 806–822, doi: 10.1080/07075332.1998.9640841

Clarke, S., & Garner, S. (2010). *White Identities a Critical Sociological Approach*. Pluto Press: London, UK.

Condliffe, B. (2001). Racism in nursing: a critical realist approach. *Nursing Times*, **97**, 2, 40. Available at: https://www.nursingtimes.net/roles/nurse-managers/racism-in-nursing-a-critical-realist-approach-09-08-2001/

Cox, G., Sobrany, S., Jenkins, E., & Musipa, C. (2021). Will nurse leaders help eradicate 'hair racism' from nursing and health services? *Journal of Nursing Management*, Early View. https://doi-org.ezproxy.mdx.ac.uk/10.1111/jonm.13286

Crenshaw, K. (1991). Mapping the margins: intersectionality, identity politics, and violence against women of color. *Stanford Law Review*, 43, 6, 1241–1299.

Cunningham, B. M., & Scarlato, A. S. M. (2018). Ensnared by colorblindness: discourse on health care disparities. *Ethnicity and Disease*, **28**, Suppl. 1, 235–240. doi: 10.18865/ed.28.S1.235

Dangerfield, A., Ferrante, J., Jennings, K., & Moorley, C. (2020). Practical action: the way forward to eliminating racially biased treatment of BAME nurses. *Nursing in Critical Care*, **25**, 376–378. doi: 10.1111.nicc.12568i

DiAngelo, R. (2018). *White Fragility*. London: Penguin Random House UK.

Dreger, A. (2015). *Galileo's Middle Finger, Heretics, Activists and One Scholar's Search for Justice*. London: Penguin Books.

Drevdahl, D., Philips, D. A., & Taylor, J. Y. (2006). Uncontested categories: the use of race and ethnicity variables in nursing research. *Nursing Inquiry*, **13**, 1, 52–63. doi: 10.1111/j.1440-1800.2006.00305.x

Equality and Human Rights Commission. (2016). Healing a Divided Britain: the need for a comprehensive race equality strategy. https://www.equalityhumanrights.com/sites/default/files/healing_a_divided_britain_-_the_need_for_a_comprehensive_race_equality_strategy_final.pdf

European Union. (2015). Discrimination in the EU in 2015. https://www.archive.equineteurope.org/IMG/pdf/ebs_437_sum_en.pdf

Evans, K., Guile, D., Harris, J., & Allan, H. T. (2010). Putting knowledge to work: a new approach. *Nurse Education Today*, 30 3, 245–251.

Flanigan, A., Frey, T., Stacy, L., & Christiansen, M. A. (2021). Updated guidance on the reporting of race and ethnicity in medical and science journals. *Journal of American Medical Association*, **326** 7, 621–627. https://jamanetwork.com/ on 09/20/202121

Foster, S. (2020). BAME staff and microaggressions. *British Journal of Nursing*, **29**, 13, 797. Available at: https:www.magonlinelibrary.com by 158.094.254.101

Frankenberg, R. (1994). *The Social Construction of Whiteness: White Women, Race Matters*. Minneapolis: University of Minnesota Press.

Fraser, S. (1995). *The Bell Curve Wars: Race, Intelligence, and the Future of America*. New York: Basic Books.

Garner, S. (2007). *Whiteness: An Introduction*. London: Routledge.

Garner, S. (2009). Empirical research into white racialized identities in Britain. *Sociology Compass*, **3**, 5, 789–802.

Giddens, A. 1(984). *Sociology*, 5th edition. Cambridge: Polity Press.

Grumbling Appendix. (2016). *Radical Nurses Archive. A Record of British Nurse Activism in the 1980s*. Available at: https://radicalnursesarchive.wordpress.com/

Hackett, R. A., Ronaldson, A., Bhui, K., et al. (2020). Racial discrimination and health: a prospective study of ethnic minorities in the United Kingdom. *BMC Public Health*, **20**, 1652. https://doi.org/10.1186/s12889-020-09792-1

Hall, J. M., & Fields, B. (2012). Continuing the conversation in nursing on race and racism. *Nursing Outlook*, **61**, 3, 164–173. https://doi. org/10.1016/j.outlo ok.2012.11.006

Hall, J. M., & Fields, B. (2013). Continuing the conversation in nursing on race and racism. *Nursing Outlook*, **61**, 3, 164–173. doi. org/10.1016/j.outlo ok.2012.11.006

Hilario, C., Browne. A. J., & McFadden, A. (2017). The influence of democratic racism in nursing inquiry. *Nursing Inquiry*, e12213. https://doi.org/10.1111/nin.12213

Holland, A. E. (2015). The lived experience of teaching about race in cultural nursing education. *Journal of Transcultural Nursing*, **26**, 1. doi: 10.1177/1043659614523995

Iheduru-Anderson, K., Shingles, R. R., & Akanegbu, C. (2021). Discourse of race and racism in nursing: an integrative review of literature. *Public Health Nursing*, **38**, 1, 115–130. https://doi.org/10.1111/phn.12828

Lamont, M. (2000). *The Dignity of Working Men.* Cambridge, MA: Harvard University Press.

Larsen, J., Allan, H. T., Bryan, K., & Smith, P. (2005). Overseas' nurses' motives for working in the UK: global perspectives or local prejudice. *Work, Employment & Society*, **19**, 2, 349–368. https://doi.org/10.1177/0950017005053177

Lebron, C. (2017). *The Making of Black Lives Matter: A Brief History of an Idea.* New York: Oxford University Press.

Likupe, G., & Archibong, U. E. (2013). Black African nurses' experiences of equality, racism, and discrimination in the National Health Service. *Journal of Psychological and Organizational Culture*, **3**, 227–246.

Lippert-Rasmussen, K. (2006). The badness of discrimination. *Ethical Theory and Moral Practice*, **9**, 2, 167–185.

Kelley, N., Khan, O., & Sharrock, S. (2017). *Racial Prejudice in Britain Today.* London: NatCen Social Research and Runnymede Trust.

Kendi, I. (2020). TED talk. https://www.youtube.com/watch?v=KCxbl5QgFZw

Kinnair, D. (2020, June 9). Beyond Covid-19, we need action and investment to address systemic inequality in our health and care systems. *Royal College of Nursing*.

Kline, R. (2014). 'The snowy white peaks' of the NHS: a survey of discrimination in governance and leadership and the potential impact on patient care in London and England. Middlesex University Repository. Monograph. Doi: http://doi.org/10.22023/mdx.12640421.v1. http://eprints.mdx.ac.uk

Kline, R. (2020, June 13). After the speeches: what now for NHS staff race discrimination? by Roger Kline. *BMJ Leader*. Retrieved from https://blogs.bmj.com/bmjleader/2020/06/13/after-the-speeches-whatnow-for-nhs-staff-race-discrimination-by-roger-kline/?utm_campaign=shareaholic&utm_medium=twitter&utm_source=socialnetwork

Knight, M., Bunch, K., Kenyon, S., Tuffnell, D., & Kurinczuk, J. J. (2020). A national population-based cohort study to investigate inequalities in maternal mortality in the United Kingdom, 2009-17. *Paediatr Perinat Epidemiol*, **34**, 392–398. https://doi.org/10.1111/ppe.12640

Kushnick, L. (1988). Racism, the national health service, and the health of black people. *International Journal of Health Services*, **18**, 3, 457–470. doi: 10.2190/LEUW-X7VW-Q2KD-UML9

McKay, J. (2020). Nurses protest in support of Black Lives Matter. Available at: https://nursingnotes.co.uk/news/workforce/nurses-protest-support-black-lives-matter/

Marmot, M., Allen, J., Boyce, T., Goldblatt, P., & Morrison, J. (2020). *Health Equity in England: The Marmot Review 10 Years On.* Institute of Health Equity. health.org.uk/publications/reports/the-marmot-review-10-years-on

Miles, R., & Brown, M. (2003). *Racism* (2nd ed.). London: Routledge.

Mitchell, A., Koch, T., & Allan, H. T. (2017). 'It's a *Touch of Sugar*': Guyanese women's beliefs about diabetes. *Action Research Journal*, **18**, 4, 433–447. https://doi.org/10.1177/1476750317721303

Moorley, C., Darbyshire, P., Serrant, L., Mohamed, J., Ali, P., & De Souza, R. (2020). Dismantling structural racism: Nursing must not be caught on the wrong side of history. *Journal of Advanced Nursing*, **76**, 10, 2450–2453.

Nayak, A. (2007). Critical whiteness studies. *Sociology Compass*, 1, 2, 737–755.

Olusanya, B. O. (2021). Systemic racism in global health: a personal reflection. *Lancet*, 9, 8, E1051–E1052. doi: 10.1016/S2214-109X(21)00147-9.051-

Olusoga, D. (2016). *Black and British: A Forgotten History*. Oxford: MacMillan.

Pan, D., Szec, S., Minhasc, J. S., Bangashd, M. S., Pareekf, N., Divallg, P., Williams, C. M. L., Oggionih, M. R., Squire, I. B., Nellumsi, L. B., Hanifj, W., Khuntik, K., & Pareeka, M. (2020). The impact of ethnicity on clinical outcomes in COVID-19: A systematic review. *The Lancet*, 3. https://doi.org/10.1016/j.eclinm.2020.100404

Public Health England. (2020). Disparities in the risk and outcomes of COVID-19. Publishing.service.gov.uk

Puzan, E. (2003). The unbearable whiteness of being (in nursing). *Nursing Inquiry*, 10, 3, 193–200. https://doi.org/10.1046/j.1440-1800.2003.00180.x

Reynolds, D. (2019). *Island Stories: Britain and Its History in the Age of Brexit*. London: Harper Collins Publishers.

Rollock, N. (2022). *The Racial Code: Tales of Reistance and Survival*. London: Penguin Random House.

Saini, A. (2019). *Superior: The Return of Race Science*. Beacon Press.

Skibba, R. (2019). The disturbing resilience of scientific racism. *Smithsonian Magazine*. https://www.smithsonianmag.com/science-nature/disturbing-resilience-scientific-racism-180972243/

Smith, P. A., Allan, H. T., Larsen, J. A., Henry, L., & MacKintosh, M. M. (2008). *Valuing and Recognising the Talents of a Diverse Healthcare Workforce*. Available at: http://www.rcn.org.uk/__data/assets/pdf_file/0008/78713/003078.pdf

Snee, H., & Goswami, H. (2020). Who cares? Social mobility and the 'class ceiling' in nursing. *Sociological Research Inline*, 26, 3, 562–580. https://doi.org/10.1177/1360780420971657

Solomos, J. (2020). Foreword from the BSA President, in Joseph-Salisbury, R., Ashe, S., Alexander, C., & Campion, K. (Eds.), *Race and ethnicity in British sociology*. Retrieved from: https://es.britsoc.co.uk/bsaCommentary/wp-content/uploads/2020/06/BSA_race_and_ethnicity_in_british_sociology_report_pre_publication_version.pdf

Stake-Doucet, N. (2020). Beyond Florence. The racist lady with the lamp. *Nursing Clio*, November 5, 2020. Available at: https://nursingclio.org/2020/11/05/the-racist-lady-with-the-lamp/

Stollznow, K. (2021). Why is it offensive to say 'all lives matter'? *The Conversation*. Available at: https://theconversation.com/why-is-it-so-offensive-to-say-all-lives-matter-153188

The Equality Act. (2010). https://www.legislation.gov.uk/ukpga/2010/15/contents

The Race Relations Act. (1968). https://www.legislation.gov.uk/ukpga/1968/71/enacted

Thorne, S. (2020). Pandemic racism – and the nursing response. *Nursing Inquiry*, 27, 3, e12371.

Thurman, W. A., Johnson, K. E., & Sumpter, D. (2019). Words matter: an integrative review of institutionalized racism in nursing literature. *Advances in Nursing Science*, 42, 2, 89–108.

UK Government. (2021). Writing about ethnicity. https://www.ethnicity-facts-figures.service.gov.uk/style-guide/writing-about-ethnicity#bame-and-bme

Van Herk, K. A., Smith, D., & Andrew, C. (2011). Examining our privileges and oppressions: incorporating an intersectionality paradigm into nursing. *Nursing Inquiry*, **18**, 1, 29–39. https://doi.org/10.1111/j.1440-1800.2011.00539.x

Williams, M. T., Skinta, M. D., Kanter, J. W., et al. (2020). A qualitative study of microaggressions against African Americans on predominantly White campuses. *BMC Psychol*, **8**, 111. https://doi.org/10.1186/s40359-020-00472-8

Zack, N. (2002). *Philosophy of Science and Race*. New York: Routledge.

2 Doctoral research

The personal is academic

Michael Traynor

Introduction

In this chapter, we will explore the choices made by doctoral students regarding the topics of their theses and the methodologies that they adopt. Doctoral students in nursing tend to start their advanced studies later in life than those in many other disciplines and bring a great deal of life and working experience to their choice of study. Because of this, it is not unusual that their work has a strong autobiographical strand. Their work can also tell a story of an awakening and raising of consciousness shaped by the structure of the doctoral journey and the theoretical perspectives that they learn to bring to bear onto personal experience. Students often choose a research methodology that they feel allows the foregrounding of personal experience—that of their research participants or their own. These methods tend to take various forms of qualitative approach such as different kinds of phenomenology and narrative work.

We will also use this chapter to reflect on the experiences of supervising such work, often across differences in 'race' and sometimes gender. As the supervisors of the research around which the book is organised, we draw on DiAngelo's argument in illuminating the problem of a 'good/bad' binary position for white academics in nursing. We will address positioning ourselves in the research field as white supervisors with black or brown doctoral candidates and the complex interplay of racialised identities, as well as power dynamics in the research and supervisory processes. We will discuss the relationship between structural domination of whiteness as it intersects with the potential of individual critique and reflexivity.

Choices of topic made by doctoral students in nursing

Doctoral research undertaken by nurses in university departments of nursing in the UK has a relatively short history. Many nurses have and still continue to undertake doctoral work with supervision within cognate disciplines, popular among these being sociology and psychology. The first nursing PhD in the UK was awarded to Audrey John in 1960. Her thesis looked at the role of psychiatric nurses. The second was conferred a year later on Margaret Scott

DOI: 10.4324/9781003269915-2

Wright (later to become the first Professor of Nursing in the UK). Her work examined the performance of student nurses (Kelly et al. 2018). We believe that Professor Dame Elizabeth Nneka Anionwu, who received her doctorate in 1988, was the first black nurse to be awarded a PhD in the UK. The academic department within which doctoral work by nurses is done and, crucially, awarded is perhaps of more significance to the profession as a whole than it is to the individual student. At a disciplinary level, the award of PhDs represents a certain coming of age.

Research that one of us was involved in (Traynor and Rafferty 1998) looking at the number of PhDs completed by nurses on nursing topics between 1976 and 1993 (with a search strategy designed to detect work completed in departments outside nursing) identified just 16 completions in 1976/77 rising to 41 in the years 1992/93 and a total number of nursing PhDs of 283 completed by 1995. As the great majority of the authors of these theses lodged copies of their work in the RCN's Steinberg Collection, held in its library in Cavendish Square, it was possible to look at virtually all the nursing theses without moving from your seat! PhD awards were very much associated with a small number of well-established university departments, notably those at Edinburgh and Manchester. Currently there are 1,253 theses in the Steinberg collection and a simple search for 'nursing' theses lodged in the UK British Library reveals 1,079 at the time of writing (January 2022).[1]

In terms of PhD topic, the largest group we identified in that study examined 'the organisation of service and administrative issues' followed by those looking at 'workforce characteristics and industrial relations' while 'specific clinical problems' made up the third largest group. Although slightly awkward, this categorisation of topics results from the disciplines in which these doctorates were supervised—social sciences rather than clinical medicine. Nurses' lack of power in the clinic also meant that research on patient populations led by nurses was unlikely to happen in the early days, at least until the arrival of Nursing Development Units in the late 1980s. A related survey that we also carried out at that time (the late 1990s) looking at published nursing research (Rafferty et al. 2000) revealed publication characteristics very different to biomedical research as a whole. The great majority of published nursing research was unfunded—or rather did not declare any funding—and written by single authors employed in universities. Comparing similar time periods, the mid 1970s and the mid-1990s, showed a slight trend towards funded and team-authored work, making it more similar to comparator biomedical research. Many saw the earlier characteristics as evidence of an immature, developing research culture in nursing. In the mid-1990s, as now, there are widespread assumptions that nursing research based on clinical trials represents the norm which should be facilitated in the profession and better funded (Chief Nursing Officer for England 2021). Sometimes these clinical trials might include the measurement of outcomes that emphasise patient experience and hence address a characteristic nursing concern. In the UK, the National Institute for Health Research has a strategy to promote the involvement and visibility of nurses involved in clinical research (https://www.nihr.ac.uk/health-and-care-professionals/career-development/nurses-and-midwives.htmsquire) and provides financial support in its doctoral award schemes. However then, as now, the argument needs to be made that the strength and interest of work that goes under the label of nursing research is its diversity and eclecticism. Although two of the studies included in this book address patient-focussed issues, none of the work here could be described as a clinical trial. However, all of the studies address urgent issues for the profession, and for society at large.

Observation suggests that nurses chose topics to pursue at doctoral level that are close to their hearts. These tend to reflect either their personal biography or a work-based experience, perhaps the inkling of a hidden problem or a repeated sense that something could be done better. The workplace for nurses in the UK tends to be either the care delivery setting or the site of nurse education—university departments. Coupled with the fact that doctoral study in nursing is often undertaken alongside part-time or full-time employment, it is little surprise that much research done by nurses is done by those employed in universities and focuses on an aspect of learning and teaching or student experience. The work gathered here straddles care delivery in the NHS focussing on discrimination and outcomes, careers in the NHS and in universities and the experiences of a section of nursing students. In every case, its author has first-hand experience of the issue they are investigating. The authors bring together a doctoral student's curiosity with a desire to examine and expose an injustice and, from the viewpoint of a supervisor, each has, whether they intended to or not at the outset, ended up exploring their own biography and identity. An alternative, perhaps you might say more 'conventional' approach to doctoral research is to become interested in a topic through coming across it in the literature and then spend the most part of the first year negotiating access to the field. In contrast, the contributors to this book are already in the field. They live it and breathe it. Their challenge has been, not to get into the field but to get away from it. Getting away means not only claiming the time from busy jobs to write and to think and collect data but also to develop the ability to forge a critical distance from the concerns and assumptions of the various fields that they are immersed in. We will discuss the value associated with 'distance' towards the end of this chapter.

Racism on the agenda

As we have pointed out in the previous pages, there is more to the origin of the studies included in this book than the personal. The authors can talk about this in their own chapters better than we can. The topic that unites their work—racism—is political on a global scale and it acts in different ways

> Racism is both overt and covert. It takes two, closely related forms: individual whites acting against individual blacks, and acts by the total

white community against the black community. We call these individual racism and institutional racism. The first consists of overt acts by individuals, which cause death, injury or the violent destruction of property. This type can be recorded by television cameras; it can frequently be observed in the process of commission. The second type is less overt, far more subtle, less identifiable in terms of specific individuals committing the acts. But it is no less destructive of human life. The second type originates in the operation of established and respected forces in the society, and thus receives far less public condemnation than the first type.

(Ture and Hamilton 1992, p. 1)

This quotation from Stokely Carmichael and Charles Hamilton's 1967 book *Black Power* marks the first time that the term institutional racism was used. Since then its existence in the powerful institutions of the UK has been denied (Scarman 1981), acknowledged (McPherson 1999) and denied again (Sewell 2021). For the most part, the contributors to this book investigate institutional racism in health care and higher education. They ask, for example, what are the experiences of black nurse academics and black senior NHS managers trying to develop their careers? All of these doctoral projects work in already established fields of inquiry though some fields are more developed than others. In the NHS, workforce issues and barriers to promotion experienced by employees from black and ethnic minority background have been both the subject of research (Kline 2014) and of many NHS initiatives such as the Workforce Race Equality Standard set up in 2015 (see https://www.england.nhs.uk/about/equality/equality-hub/equality-standard/). These are examples taken from two of the topics that appear in this book. So, we can locate the work of these doctoral candidates as operating within and contributing to a policy landscape and see the combination of the personal and the political in their projects.

Where do we find theory and method?

But accounts of personal experience, whether the experiences of research participants or the candidates' own, though central, are not sufficient to make a PhD or professional doctorate. The essential feature of doctoral work is the understanding of 'data'—in the case of much of the work included here this takes the form of accounts of experience—within a theoretical framework. At the risk of rehearsing an over-familiar argument, the need for theory is not just in order to fill out a methods chapter or to write seemingly obligatory passages about epistemology and ontology to satisfy examiners. 'Data', even the apparently 'authentic' experiences of research participants, or 'objective' workforce statistics never speak for themselves. That we might ever think that they do shows that we are informally applying some system of values and interpretive structure to what we see, hear and read.[2] Where do these informal systems and structures come from? Some will come from our social and personal biography but, in research which examines the way that institutions work, much will be shaped by occupational values and assumptions, both formal and highly informal. We may be so thoroughly immersed in these that they have long ago become 'natural', simply how things are. This is why grappling with theory—which challenges the natural—can be so difficult. It is because theory can transform the way that we think or rather *needs* to transform the way that we think. It is not a matter of cognitively understanding an argument that we come across in the literature or a system of assertions made by authors. Critical social theories in particular can be both transformative and counter-intuitive. They have to start to transform the way we think while we are still thinking in the old, untransformed, way. Students, or anyone, discovering critical race theory or post-structuralist theory about human subjectivity, to take two examples, have to journey far enough into an experience of non-comprehension to start to find glimmers of something exciting going on. The first glimmer might be recognising certain forms of argument, or certain concerns or debates, or the recurrence of key ideas by certain writers. The sense of bewilderment and annoyance might start to ease slightly as the discoverer of theory starts to ask, 'So supposing for a moment that this is true, what might it mean for my work—and for my thinking?' This journey demands both hard work and courage. Any desire to be shot of the PhD does not help. Intellectual courage is needed, even as a thought experiment, to cut the ties to our particular form of common sense or occupational thinking and give credence to a new way of seeing the world. A failure at this point might take the form of holding on to our ingrained way of thinking and attempting to fit this new theory we are reading about somehow inside it. For example, we might like what we read in sociological theories of occupational closure when applied to medicine but it is only when we realise that these theories also apply to our own profession that the true transformation by theory can occur. This can be either a moment of utter excitement or the moment when we turn back and fake it for the examiners. Thinking, though, about the example we chose of critical race theory, it could well be that the experience that a new reader has in this field might not be one of bewilderment but of, possibly sudden, recognition. See the next section.

So, to backtrack a little, theory or a theoretical framework enables a crucial noticing, or perhaps rather a creating of patterns within data. It suggests a way to bring different elements together and, if it is possible to say this, to explain what is happening. It provides a structure for thinking about the data and for writing about it and, ultimately, a structure and approach for the whole thesis, a perspective. Far from being a time-consuming add-on to doctoral work, theory is the key that allows everything to fall into place. And because theory, by definition, develops at a high level of generalisation, its use enables our findings to be put in the context of other findings from possibly very different settings. It enables our work to take its place alongside other work in this field and it can place the doctoral student in the community of workers within that field.

Theory as consciousness-raising

Most people see the idea of consciousness-raising as originating from within the women's movement of the late 1960s and 1970s along with black consciousness movements of a similar time, although the term owes something to Marxist ideas about liberation from the false consciousness of ideology. Groups of women would meet to discuss the problems that they faced as individuals and by discussion with others come to the realisation that their problems were not individual failures at all but examples of patriarchy in action. In other words, their experiences and frustrations were the result of highly generalised structural features of societies across the globe.

As one participant says in a reflection of membership of one of those groups:

> ...women didn't understand why they felt so bad, they didn't understand why they were so... they really couldn't do the things they wanted to do, it was just a kind of terrible mystery. So it's only by talking about it that there began to be some understanding and it was really understanding about oppression and where does the oppression come from and who's oppressing me and how can this be overcome. You know, these really quite basic life questions women were grappling with in these consciousness-raising groups.
> (Sisterhood and After Research Team 2013)

For the doctoral students involved in this book the principles of consciousness-raising are doubly relevant. First, as a community of researchers, albeit those with other identities as lecturer, NHS worker, mother or father, their experiences as witnesses to racism and sometimes as those who share the experiences of racism that their participants describe allow them to understand the commonalities across the different groups that they are working with. Second, the discovery of theory that 'makes sense' of enigmatic and uncomfortable experience can enable a liberating moment of distance, distance both from personal suffering and from organisational and institutional priorities and imperatives. Sometimes the mere identification and naming of a phenomenon such as microaggression or white fragility can evoke a hugely helpful sense of recognition and empowerment. This empowerment in turn can become the engine for material change. That change can take the form of new personal life choices or of action to address the injustices faced by research participants or those who might take their place in the future.

Many doctoral supervisors are waiting for, and trying to create suitable conditions for, that moment from the student when they realise how theory can transform the way they approach their work.

The difference between theory and method

The kind of overarching theoretical framework that we have just been discussing needs to be distinguished from methodology. But before we do that, it is worth saying two things: the first is that these two, theory and methodology, should be interrelated in doctoral work or rather there should be a consistency between them; the second is that some methodologies around data collection and analysis have a heavy theoretical or philosophical component that can feel a lot like a sufficient theoretical framework for the whole thesis but actually is not.

Most supervisors and examiners would expect that the methods used in a thesis would reflect the overall theoretical orientation taken by its author. To explore this let's look at the example of what has become known as 'feminist research'. When feminist research first emerged researchers who were developing it wanted to eradicate any element of power differential between the researcher and the researched (Showalter 1986, Lather 1991, Benhabib et al. 1995). They associated this imbalance with patriarchy and gendered notions of (the possibility of) the detached value-free scientist. This value-free observer had access to a system of knowledge that had a greater trustworthiness than the informal knowledge that might have been associated (perhaps stereotypically) with women—embodied, intuitive. While there are a great many lists of the characteristics of feminist research, there is some consensus. One writer proposes five key features: *a gender perspective, accentuation of women's experiences, reflexivity, participatory methods, and social action* (Taylor 1998). Alongside the ethical and political features we can see methodological characteristics. This overall approach to research shares with critical race theory, which we will discuss later, an emancipatory ambition rather than an aim to impartially collect information to be used by others in decision-making positions. Its research questions start from feminist concerns that topics of importance to women have been systematically ignored by a largely male research establishment and male-centric research agenda (see Anne Oakley's research on housework (Oakley 1976)). Feminist research foregrounds the experiences and the views of women—it has been said that it 'validates' them, brings them to light or 'gives them voice', although such terms are problematic because they suggest that status differentials are still at work. Such research is reflexive because the researcher does not try to believe that they are outside the research simply collecting data but acknowledges that they are inevitably involved and influencing the work and the resulting data, and because of this they need to make efforts to become aware of their positioning and influence and write this into the work. In other words, feminist research acknowledges that it is relational. Probably most feminist researchers have been and continue to be women and its likely, given the argument just rehearsed, that they have been largely involved in interaction with female research participants. The researchers contributing to this book also have a stake in the research topics they have chosen, though not necessarily a gendered stake. Reading some of their transcripts of interviews with black academics or black NHS managers undertaken by black doctoral students, it is hard to imagine that white researcher-interviewers would have brought out such frank responses. (See their individual chapters; not all of the authors are black.) So, their method of data collection, highly participatory qualitative, sometimes narrative interviews, has a consistency with an overall emancipatory and non-hierarchical theoretical standpoint. Finally, to come full circle, feminist research is seen as a part of social action in all the ways just described as well as in its potential to bring to light injustice or oppression, and the details of their workings and first-hand accounts of their impacts and responses to them.

Khiara Bridges described critical race theory as providing an 'analytical toolset for interrogating the relationship between law and racial inequality' (Bridges 2019). The emancipatory orientation of critical race theory, like feminist research, locates this work within critical theory with its commitment to critiquing and changing society (Horkheimer 1972) rather than working within a belief in a neutrality that in effect supports the functioning of the status quo. From a feminist point of view the status quo is patriarchy and from critical race theory, white privilege and white supremacy.

Crucial to our argument here about the need for consistency but not identity between theory and method, we note that the methods often used in research within these theoretical traditions are participatory, as mentioned earlier. By 'participatory' we are not referring specifically to the procedures that go under the name of 'participatory action research', although that research approach could be considered to have emancipatory origins, rather to an approach to 'data collection' that allows the research participants to set the agenda as a more-or-less equal with the researcher. The data that emerges would typically be qualitative in nature, the result of conversations between researcher and the research participants, though there is no intrinsic correspondence between qualitative methods and feminist or critical race concerns as feminist Ann Oakley argues (Oakley 2000). Collecting survey data or analysing existing large statistical datasets can certainly be carried out with emancipatory intentions and outcome as much early British sociological research shows (Carr-Saunders et al. 1958/1927).

So, to move our argument on, we would like to suggest that while methodology needs to be consistent with an overall theoretical and epistemological commitment, it cannot be *sufficient* to provide a framework for an overarching interpretation of the 'data' collected. And if it is not obvious by now, we are placing 'data' in quotations to signal that the accounts of research participants need to be understood, not as 'given' or 'found' but as produced by the research process within which the researcher plays an unavoidably influential role. As we have already mentioned, the reason that we want to spend time on this argument is that many research methodologies have been developed and are presented as having strong theoretical founding assumptions. Those who are new to research at this level and who give a great deal of attention to methodology may well mistake the rigours of methodology for the framework that can provide meaning to their data. Probably all of the methodologies adopted by contributors here as well as many that are not included have this potential for misrecognition. Setting out just two of these methodologies—phenomenology and narrative analysis—now might make this clearer. They both work from the assumption that what people say is worth listening to but perhaps for different reasons.

Looking first at phenomenology, it will be all too clear that what is widely used today as a research methodology started out as the label for a philosophical project whose aim was to properly understand human subjective existence via an investigation of the structures of experience and consciousness. At least since Descartes and, later, Hegel, European philosophers had been focussed on the identification of a foundational science and foundational knowledge that banished all unfounded assumptions (Critchley 2001). Phenomenology needs to be understood within this context, as one development of this project. Since its early 20th century origins, approaches to this project have proliferated and diversified. Nevertheless, those learning from scratch about this broad approach are presented with a choice between two basic versions: so-called descriptive phenomenology and an 'interpretive' alternative, associated with the names of their apparent proponents, Edmund Husserl (1859–1938) and Martin Heidegger (1889–1976) respectively. Despite some key differences in starting point, both philosophers were working on developing a basic understanding of human existence and consciousness. We would like to make two points. The first is that to all intents and purposes, the phenomenological 'project' can be seen as providing both a topic and a method, the topic being the nature of consciousness and being; the method being the attempt to set aside taken-for-granted assumptions, this attempt being known as (various forms of) reduction. The second point is that an attraction of phenomenology (perhaps especially to doctoral researchers) is that it appears to offer a sufficiently strong and sophisticated theoretical foundation for broadly qualitative work involving the gathering of personal accounts and views of research participants. A problem might arise when the phenomenological project (described above) forces its way into the research objectives of the researcher who starts out wanting to understand social processes, such as racism. Phenomenology certainly foregrounds subjective experience because the nature of consciousness and experience was its original focus but it does not provide theory about the character and operation of social processes such as racism. The gravitas of its founders and the sheer time and effort required to understand their work can distract the new researcher into believing that a thorough phenomenological analysis is the end point of their analysis rather than a tool to manage their data and facilitate thinking about it. To point out this potential problem is not to underrate the usefulness of subsequent developments of phenomenological thinking. The useful impact of the phenomenological project on social research has been indirect, though fascinating. Alfred Schütz (1899–1959) a partial contemporary of both Husserl and Heidegger attempted to bring a philosophical study of subjective experience, for example the experience of time, to Max Weber's sociological theories. His work, such as his 1932 *The Phenomenology of the Social World* (Schutz 1967) has been foundational in the development of thinking in the social sciences. A sociological interest in the 'life-world' and the development of the now almost ubiquitous social constructionism both owe a great deal to Schütz, his followers and collaborators such as Thomas Luckmann and to phenomenology.

Now we turn to narrative analysis. Narrative analysis or narrative inquiry as it is often known, like phenomenological research, is undertaken by researchers in different disciplines and the term does not describe one unified practice. Broadly, and unsurprisingly, it refers to research that uses stories and storytelling as sources of knowledge. Narrative researchers are interested not only in the content of stories but in the structure that can, they argue, be detected or discovered within them. In another similarity to phenomenology, narrative inquiry, in certain hands, can be exactly what its name suggests—research into the features of stories. In other words, it supplies its own topic. American linguist William Labov (b. 1927) is renowned for work examining the linguistic features of vernacular American. Regarding narrative, he has devised a well-used six (or five) feature structure which he sees as characterising 'well-formed' narratives (Labov and Waletzky 1997). For workers in Labov's tradition any individual story is useful as an example that can help refine an understanding of the structure of stories. Before we go on to talk about more applied and sociological use of narrative inquiry we want to linger a little longer with the idea that the stories told by humans can be themselves the topic of research and theorising rather than of use primarily as windows onto a social world. Corinne Squire's introduction to *Doing Narrative Research* sets out a basic division between humanistic and structuralist approaches to narrative

> The first [influence on narrative research] is the post-war rise of humanist approaches within western social sciences. These approaches posed holistic, person-centred approaches, often including attention to individual case studies, biographies and life histories, against what they saw as positivist empiricism... The second influence on contemporary narrative research, is Russian structuralist and later, French poststructuralist (Barthes, 1977, Culler, 2002; Genette, 1979, Todorov, 1990) postmodern (Foucault, 1972; Lyotard, 1984), psychoanalytic (Lacan, 1977) and deconstructionist (Derrida, 1977) approaches to narrative within the humanities.
>
> (Squire et al. 2008, p. 7)

Squire's summary of the flavour of the latter [post-structuralist approaches to narrative] is succinct:

> ...unlike the humanist narrative... it [is] concerned with narrative fluidity and contradiction, with unconscious as well as conscious meanings, and with the power relations within which narratives become

possible... It assumed that multiple, disunified subjectivities were involved in the production and understanding of narratives, rather than singular, agentic storytellers and hearers, and it was preoccupied with the social formations shaping language and subjectivity. In this tradition, the storyteller does not tell the story, so much as s/he is told by it.

(Squire et al. 2008, p. 8)

So, the researcher whose research topic is racism and who is new to narrative work is faced with a similar predicament to the beginning phenomenological researcher. It is possible that they become so confronted by debates and complexities within theories of storytelling and subjectivity that their analysis struggles to go further than grappling with and discovering aspects of narratives told by their participants. Fortunately, as with phenomenology, there are plenty of examples of the method applied to highly contextualised social research. Catherine Kohler Riessman's work (Riessman 1993) includes both research into topics such as the impact of divorce as well as reviews of similarly applied work. The whole field of medical sociology leans heavily on the study of what have become known as 'illness narratives' (Bury 1982). To go further, its early explorers, among them Arthur Frank, Arthur Kleinman and Elliot Mishler, proposed that serious illness transforms a *person* into a *patient* moving into a territory that is colonised by the medical profession and bringing a profound sense of loss. In this tradition, the telling of a story of their illness by a 'patient' can become a critical tool not merely for a personal coming to terms with that loss but more fundamentally for resisting entrapment by medical conceptualisations (Greenhalgh 2016). To summarise, some narrative researchers are primarily concerned with advancing an understanding of narratives themselves. Others apply this approach to attempts to understand social processes, sometimes at a societal level.

At this point, we need to open a short discussion on the popular methodological approach grounded theory.[3] This is because some writers on methodology may well see grounded theory as an exception to the claims about theory that we have just outlined. They might argue that valid, generalisable, conceptual statements about data—theory we might say—can and should be discovered within the data gathered from a particular research study rather than be developed separately from it and brought to bear on, an approach that our earlier arguments have pointed to i.e. critical race theory exists 'outside' or prior to our project and we bring it to bear on our thinking and our data. At the heart of the method's development in early to mid-1960s United States, was its founders' belief that current theory in sociology had become an exercise in 'logico-deductive thinking' (Corbin 2013) rather than being based in actual data which contemporary sociology was in danger of losing touch with. There are elements of the broader debate between empiricist and rationalist philosophies at work in this dichotomy (Critchley 2001). Researchers using grounded theory typically set out to discover basic social processes in specific situations, such as how the relatives and doctors involved with dying people might try to shape their awareness of impending death (Glaser and Strauss 1965). The results of such work might be considered to be what Merton decades earlier had called 'middle-range' theory in his own effort to reground sociology and in opposition to the work of Talcott Parsons (Merton 1968) whose approach he considered remote from the empirical world. The accumulated findings of middle-range work over time, Merton argued, may well allow sociologists to propose more broad-ranging theories at some future date. Merton first made these arguments in the 1940s and 1950s, nearly 80 years ago, so we might be justified in expecting that some of these theories are available to today's researchers. We would like to suggest that the contributors to this book have approached data analysis with the detail and care that many grounded theorists would apply. A difference, perhaps, is that alongside their analysis they have explored the usefulness of existing theoretical frameworks such as that provided by critical race theory. The model here is one of iteration between close examination of data and reflection on the implications of a theoretical approach. The outcome is not only 'findings' that link the social processes found in the accounts of participants to global forces but, possibly, extensions or proposed adaptations to existing theory based on the particularity of the data.

So, to summarise this first part of this chapter, we have discussed the choices that doctoral students are faced with regarding topic, theory and methodology in their work. We now move on to look at the process of, or rather the factors that influence, supervision itself.

Supervising across 'race' and gender

Doctoral supervision, in nursing and other academic disciplines, has been examined and sometimes problematised in writing by both supervisors and students, and sometimes both together (Li and Seale 2007). Much of this work is anecdotal, written from the supervisor's viewpoint (as this is) and fails to engage with structural issues of power, race or class e.g. (Parker-Jenkins 2018, Jackson et al. 2021). Only a few studies are based on data from supervisory interactions (Cargill 2000, Li and Seale 2007). Gorup and Laufer review research, including findings from a number of large surveys, that highlights the control and sometimes abuse of power that many doctoral students, particularly those from overseas to the host institution have experienced (Gorup and Laufer 2020). Issues involve a lack of accountability for supervisors within institutions and the abuse of power by supervisors (and sometimes examiners) who may not only have control over the student's funding but their immigration status and their future career as well. An international and cross-disciplinary survey conducted by the journal Nature, referenced by Gorup and Laufer, reported that 21% of all their participants (n=6,300) reported that they had experienced discrimination or harassment in their PhD program. Of these, 39% said that they had experienced gender-based discrimination and 33% racial discrimination or harassment (Woolston 2019). There is clearly a power differential between doctoral students and supervisors that can be augmented by race and gender-based differences, particularly where overseas students are involved. And as in most fields, organisational pressures for example those on recruitment numbers and completion rates can influence the behaviour of actors in sometimes negative ways.

A review of PhD study within the social sciences by ESRC found that '[t]here is prima facie evidence of a lack of diversity' but that the topic lacked systematic comparative research on how diversity and inclusion are affected by the form of doctoral education. The model(s) of social science doctoral work and supervision is perhaps more similar to that of nursing than the frequent picture of PhD students as working in labs in large teams managed by a senior academic who also supervises the postgraduate students. The study goes on to say:

> In the limited number of UK studies of BAME doctoral students, two themes are prominent. First, BAME doctoral students report similar sets of issues as other doctoral students (in terms of financial insecurity, supervision issues, etc.), but these tend to be experienced more acutely, and as part of intersectional disadvantage (Arday, 2017; Mattocks & Briscoe-Palmer, 2016). They also report experiencing the 'institutionalised whiteness' of the academy, in common with the recurrent testimony of BAME academic staff (e.g. Bhopal et al., 2015).
>
> (CFE Research and University of York 2020, p. 33)

But the studies that identify overt and sometimes outrageous examples of abuse of supervisor power over black and ethnic minority students, though important, in some ways reinforce a white belief that racism is something that racists—other people—do. In situations where supervisors as well as examiners are white and well intentioned, students who are black or brown will quickly understand, if they did not already, that the gatekeepers to doctoral success and to an academic career are enshrined in whiteness. Whiteness is the norm in academic institutions, as it is in most others, so that it can be mistaken for transparency, for no colour at all.

What might be the implications of this? One might be that black or brown PhD students might be denied the 'luxury of impartiality' to paraphrase DiAngelo (Waldman 2018). To carry on this line of critique, impartiality, detachment and rigour would be seen to be the preserve of white people (and possibly only white men) because they are transparent and universal while black people and possibly women are characterised by being embodied deviations from this transparent norm. The assumption would be that black people or women have a race or gender-based identity that situates and limits them in a way that white people (and possibly, again, only white men) somehow do not. If white people, including white supervisors, are the beneficiaries of racism and white privilege, a doctoral student, or potential student, arriving with a project to examine the operation of racism—especially racism in the university—may well present a certain challenge. It is here that DiAngelo's 'good/bad binary' the belief held by many white people of a world peopled by evil racists and compassionate non-racists, might help the black doctoral student wishing to research racism. A liberal supervisor is likely long ago to have accepted and even championed the 'committed' or 'situated' researcher and their project so it is unlikely, though still possible, that the black or brown student proposing to research racism will be rejected at this stage. But as the supervisory practice and relationship progresses tensions and ambiguities, verbalised or not, are likely to develop. The student may feel some anxiety about holding up a mirror to white supervisors or about disclosing their own experiences of racism. The white supervisor may try to disentangle methodological concerns from their reluctance to believe in the ubiquity of the operation of racism and white privilege or be confused about whether to suggest other explanations for injustice, such as class. The student may learn to dial down their anger or their energy for the topic and adopt the white academic's tentative tone. The supervisor may read data describing overt racism with a sense of relief (because they can objectify it). Conversely the supervisor may feel frustrated that their black student seems to *not* want to name racism in their data. So, the situation of white supervisor(s)/black student unavoidably embodies race-based power relations in the university. It might though, present an opportunity for white supervisors to become aware of and reflect on their own privilege in academic institutions and in wider society. The involvement of non-white supervisors and examiners can go some way to soften the contrast but every supervisor needs to be supervising because they have relevant expertise and not because they have been invited onto the team to make white supervisors feel more 'inclusive'. The same applies to doctoral examiners.

We have already mentioned how the feminist consciousness-raising movement that emerged during the 1970s has formed a long-standing, if widely forgotten, foundation for thinking about and action on gender. Fifty years later, it seems that much has improved but simultaneously things are as bad as ever they were. The gender pay gap in the UK has shrunk from a median of 47.6% in 1970 to 16.8 in 2016 (Ward 2018) and indications are that it has fallen further since then yet many occupations such as highly rewarded engineering (88% men (Women's Engineering Society 2022)) and not so highly rewarded nursing (89% women (Nursing and Midwifery Council 2021)) remain strongly gendered. In the workplace, women continue to face barriers to promotion to senior managerial roles (Kings Fund 2013). At a different level, 30% of women worldwide have been subjected to either physical and/or sexual intimate partner violence or non-partner sexual violence in their lifetime (World Health Organization 2021) and the #MeToo movement has revealed widespread sexual abuse and harassment of women coupled with abuse of power (Wikipedia contributors 2022). Doctoral supervision across genders raises similar issues regarding power as does ethnicity and interacts with beliefs about race in complex ways, one effect being the potential for multiple, intersecting, disadvantage. That nursing is a predominantly female profession that does not face the same challenges of STEM subjects in terms of the under-representation of women, does not mean that gender is not an issue within doctoral supervision. Though approximately ten per cent of the UK nursing workforce is male, men are more highly represented in senior academic roles. The Royal College of Nursing's on-going survey of UK professors with a nursing background reveals that of the 262 professors identified across 79 institutions, 68 (26%) are men (see https://www.rcn.org.uk/professional-development/research-and-innovation/research-training-and-careers/the-nursing-professoriate-in-the-uk). They are overrepresented as first authors on research papers in nursing journals particularly in UK-based journals (Shields et al. 2011). A common attribution for this difference is the different involvement in family caring work that men and women take up and are expected to take up. In fact, Lindhardt and Berthelsen suggest that many of those female nursing academics who have been successful have 'sacrificed' what is usually considered as the satisfactions of family and social life for a focus on work (Lindhardt and Berthelsen 2017). So doctoral students in nursing are perhaps rather more likely to encounter male supervisors. Returning to the concept of intersectionality, the argument is that, for example, a black woman working, or studying in our case, in a context where white men predominate, or dominate by having set up the rules, is likely to face two levels of structural inequality that interact in ways that make it different in character to that which might be experienced by a black man or a white woman. The notion of intersectionality was originally developed in the context of and as a challenge to discrimination in the US legal system (Crenshaw 1989) i.e. structural disadvantage but has broadened into a way of understanding individual experiences of discrimination and disadvantage and has become a touchstone for controversy within US culture wars (Gray 2018). Despite the recent high visibility of the term and the debate surrounding it, many feminists at least since the 1980s, if not long before, had been arguing that the essentialist term 'woman' covered over a multiplicity of identities and positions of varying privilege and disadvantage (see Nicholson (1990) for a fascinating collection of essays debating feminism and postmodernism). The power differentials at play within doctoral supervision, then, have to be understood in terms of intersectionality, not solely in terms of gender differences nor of differences in ethnicity. Individual supervisor/student teams may have established what they feel to be collegiate, friendly and non-hierarchical working relationships but, desirable as this approach is, structural power differentials remain—and are perhaps more obvious to students than they are to supervisors.

The six doctoral contributors to this book can be described as follows: three are women, three are men; of the men two are black and one is white; all of the women are black. Supervisors: Helen Allan acts as supervisor for five of the contributors; Michael Traynor is involved with two of them (MO and DS). Both of us are white. The supervisory teams also include six other colleagues who are identified in Chapter 1. Of these, four are women and two are men and three are white.

Available resources

It needs to be acknowledged, of course, that institutions—universities, trades unions and other organisations—take action and develop policies designed to reveal and combat racist, sexist and other forms of discriminatory behaviour. We have mentioned some of these initiatives and associated literature at the end of Chapter 1. In addition, universities and colleges are exploring various approaches to decolonise their curricula (see Stone and Ashton 2021). That these issues are debated at all is a sign of change but where issues of power exist, there will be resistance (by those who benefit from power) and struggle. We hope that the work of the contributors to this book becomes a resource to further that change.

Summary

In this second of two introductory chapters, we first set out a background to doctoral work done by nurses in terms of the topics and methodologies chosen. We also argued that it is important for doctoral students to engage with and be transformed by theory. We then went on to explore some of the issues of power that are at work in the practice of supervision. We focussed particularly on how ethnicity and gender can add to a complex matrix of power differentials between students and their supervisors. The next six chapters are given to the on-going work of five doctoral candidates who are each researching different aspects of racism.

Notes

1 http://explore.bl.uk/primo_library/libweb/action/search.do?srt=date&srtChange=true&frbg=&rfnGrpCounter=1&vl(488279563UI0)=any&indx=1&fn=search&dscnt=1&scp.scps=scope:(BLCONTENT)&tb=t&fctV=theses&mode=Basic&vid=BLVU1&ct=facet&rfnGrp=1&srt=rank&tab=local_tab&fctN=facet_rtype&dum=true&vl(freeText0)=Nursing&dstmp=1531225546662
2 The argument we are setting out here might be considered 'interpretive'.
3 The method's popularity in nursing research reflects the fact that its founders were employed in a school of nursing (at the University of California, San Francisco) at the time of its development (Stern 2013). For two accounts of the uptake of grounded theory in nursing departments see the consecutive chapters by Corbin (referenced above in the main text) and by Stern. The chapters are contrasting not only in their degree of personal identification with and defence of the method but in their personal presentation. Juliet Corbin writes about herself in the third person while Phyllis is very much present in her text.

References

Benhabib, S., J. P. Butler, D. Cornell and N. Fraser (1995). *Feminist Contentions: A Philosophical Exchange*. New York, Routledge.

Bridges, K. M. (2019). *Critical Race Theory: A Primer*. St. Paul, MN, Foundation Press.

Bury, M. (1982). "Chronic illness as biographical disruption." *Sociology of Health and Illness* 4: 167–182.

Cargill, M. (2000). "Intercultural postgraduate supervision meetings: an exploratory discourse study." *Prospect* 15(2): 28–38.

Carr-Saunders, A., D. Jones and C. Moser (1958/1927). *A Survey of Social Conditions in England and Wales as Illustrated in Statistics*. Oxford, Oxford University Press, originally published in 1927 as A survey of the social structure of England and Wales as illustrated in statistics.

CFE Research and University of York (2020). *Review of the PhD in Social Sciences: Rapid Evidence Assessment*. Interim report by CFE Research and University of York for the ESRC Review of the PhD in Social Sciences. Leicester, CFE Research.

Chief Nursing Officer for England (2021). *Making Research Matter Chief Nursing Officer for England's Strategic Plan for Research Version 2, November 2021*. London, NHS England and NHS Improvement.

Corbin, J. (2013). Strauss'grounded theory. In C. T. Beck (Ed.), *Routledge International Handbook of Qualitative Nursing Research*. London, Routledge: 169–182.

Crenshaw, K. (1989). *Demarginalizing the Intersection of Race and Sex: A Black Feminist Critique of Antidiscrimination Doctrine, Feminist Theory and Antiracist Politics (PDF)*. University of Chicago Legal Forum. Archived (PDF) from the original on 13 May 2018. Retrieved 7 June 2020., University of Chicago.

Critchley, S. (2001). *Continental Philosophy. A Very Short Introduction*. Oxford, Oxford University Press.

Glaser, B. and A. Strauss (1965). *The Awareness of Dying*. Chicago, IL, Aldine.

Gorup, M. and M. Laufer (2020). *More Than a Case of a Few Bad Apples: When Relationships Between Supervisors and Doctoral Researchers Go Wrong*. Retrieved 27th January, 2022, from https://elephantinthelab.org/when-relationships-between-supervisors-and-doctoral-researchers-go-wrong/

Gray, P. W. (2018). "'The fire rises': identity, the alt-right and intersectionality." *Journal of Political Ideologies* 23(2): 141–156.

Greenhalgh, T. (2016). Cultural Contexts of Health: The Use of Narrative Research in the Health Sector [Internet]. *Health Evidence Network Synthesis Report, No. 49*. Copenhagen, WHO Regional Office for Europe.

Horkheimer, M. (1972). Traditional and critical theory. *Critical Theory Selected Essays*. New York, Seabury Press.

Jackson, D., T. Power and K. Usher (2021). "Understanding doctoral supervision in nursing: 'It's a complex fusion of skills'." *Nurse Education Today* (1532-2793 (Electronic)): 1–7.

Kelly, D., L. Pollock, S. Rodgers, T. N. Fawcett and P. Smith (2018). "Leaps in the dark: 60 years of Nursing Studies at the University of Edinburgh." *Journal of Advanced Nursing* 74(1): 1–4.

Kings Fund (2013). "Women continue to face barriers to taking senior leadership positions in the NHS, new research finds." *Press Releases*. http://www.kingsfund.org.uk/press/press-releases/women-continue-face-barriers-taking-senior-leadership-positions-nhs-new 2015

Kline, R. (2014). *The "Snowy White Peaks" of the NHS: A Survey of Discrimination in Governance and Leadership and the Potential Impact on Patient Care in London and England.* Available from Middlesex University's Research Repository. Middlesex University.

Labov, W. and J. Waletzky (1997). "Narrative analysis: oral versions of personal experience." *Journal of Narrative & Life History* 7(1–4): 3–38.

Lather, P. (1991). *Getting Smart. Feminist Research and Pedagogy With/in the Postmodern.* London, Routledge.

Li, S. and C. Seale (2007). "Managing criticism in Ph.D. supervision: a qualitative case study." *Studies in Higher Education* 32(4): 511–526.

Lindhardt, T. and C. B. Berthelsen (2017). "h-index or G-spot: Female nursing researchers' conditions for an academic career." *Journal of Advanced Nursing* 73(6): 1249–1250.

McPherson, W. (1999). *The Stephen Lawrence Inquiry Report of an inquiry by Sir William Macpherson.* London, UK Home Office.

Merton, R. K. (1968). *Social Theory and Social Structure* (1968 enlarged ed.). New York, Free Press.

Nicholson, L., Ed. (1990). *Feminism/Postmodernism.* London, Routledge.

Nursing and Midwifery Council (2021). *The NMC Register Mid-year Update 1 April–30 September 2021.* London, NMC.

Oakley, A. (1976). *The Sociology of Housework.* London, Martin Robertson.

Oakley, A. (2000). *Experiments in Knowing: Gender and Method in the Social Sciences.* Cambridge, Polity Press.

Parker-Jenkins, M. (2018). "Mind the gap: developing the roles, expectations and boundaries in the doctoral supervisor–supervisee relationship." *Studies in Higher Education* 43(1): 57–71.

Rafferty, A. M., M. Traynor and G. Lewison (2000). *Measuring the Outputs of Nursing R&D: A Third Working Paper.* London, Centre for Policy in Nursing Research; London School of Hygiene & Tropical Medicine.

Riessman, C. K. (1993). *Narrative Analysis.* Newbury Park, CA, Sage.

Scarman, L. J. (1981, April 10–12). *The Brixton Disorders.* London, HMSO.

Schutz, A. (1967). *The Phenomenology of the Social World.* Evanston, Northwestern University Press.

Sewell, T. (2021). *Commission on Race and Ethnic Disparities: The Report.* London, UK Cabinet Office.

Shields, L., A. A. Hall J. Fau-Mamun and A. A. Mamun (2011). "The 'gender gap' in authorship in nursing literature." *Journal of the Royal Society of Medicine* 104(11): 457–464.

Showalter, E. (1986). Introduction: the feminist critical revolution. In E. Showalter (Ed.), *The New Feminist Criticism: Essays on Women, Literature and Theory.* London, Virago Press: 3–17.

Sisterhood and After Research Team (2013). "Consciousness raising." *Sisterhood and After.* Retrieved January 13, 2022, from https://www.bl.uk/sisterhood/articles/consciousness-raising

Squire, C., M. Andrews and M. Tamboukou (2008). What is narrative research? In M. Andrews, C. Squire and M. Tsamboukou (Eds.), *Doing Narrative Research.* London, Sage: 1–26.

Stern, P. N. (2013). Glaserian grounded theory. In C. T. Beck (Ed.), *Routledge International Handbook of Qualitative Nursing Research.* London, Routledge: 162–168.

Stone, R. V. and S. Ashton. (2021, 07/04/2021). "How not to decolonise your curriculum." Retrieved February 10, 2022, from https://wonkhe.com/blogs/how-not-to-decolonise-your-curriculum/

Taylor, V. (1998). "Feminist methodology in social movements research." *Qualitative Sociology* **21**(4): 357–379.

Traynor, M. and A. M. Rafferty (1998). *Nursing, Research and the Higher Education Context*. Centre for Policy in Nursing Research, London School of Hygiene & Tropical Medicine.

Ture, K. and C. V. Hamilton (1992). *Black Power; The Politics of Liberation in America*. New York, Vintage books.

Waldman, K. (2018). A sociologist examines the "White Fragility" that prevents White Americans from confronting racism. *The New Yorker*. New York.

Ward, D. (2018). "The gender pay gap: what now?" Retrieved February 9, 2022, from https://www.kingsfund.org.uk/blog/2018/06/gender-pay-gap-what-now?

Wikipedia Contributors (2022). "MeToo movement." Retrieved February 9, 2022, from https://en.wikipedia.org/w/index.php?title=MeToo_movement&oldid=1069816735

Women's Engineering Society (2022). "Useful statistics." Retrieved February 9, 2022, from https://www.wes.org.uk/content/wesstatistics

Woolston, C. (2019). "PhD poll reveals fear and joy, contentment and anguish." *Nature* **575**: 403–406.

World Health Organization (2021). "Violence against women." *Fact sheets*. Retrieved February 9, 2022, from https://www.who.int/news-room/fact-sheets/detail/violence-against-women

3   On listening to migrant women

Ann Mitchell

Introduction

This chapter gives voice to a group of Guyanese women who participated in a participatory action research (PAR) inquiry to share their experiences of living with Type 2 diabetes as part of a PhD study from 2010 to 2015. The women who came from different backgrounds and careers emigrated to England over 40 years ago where they faced racist issues and oppressive practices when trying to access health care for their diabetes. As a Guyanese immigrant, I recognised the issues facing them and felt uniquely privileged to be researching collaboratively with this group of women. We worked together on a process based on sharing, listening, and reconstructing stories. This study is based on Koch and Kralik's (2006) participatory action research (PAR) methodology which resonates with the key issues.

Context

Guyana, a former British colony, is the only English-speaking country in South America and a similar geographical size to Great Britain. Although linked with the English-speaking Caribbean, Guyana has its own culture and traditions due to its diverse and racially mixed population comprising Indian, African, Portuguese, Chinese, Mixed, and Indigenous heritage (Green & Emanuel 2000). The country was an important contributor to the influx of "West Indian" immigration to the UK commonly referred to as the "Windrush Generation".

Many Guyanese migrated to the UK because the British Nationality Act of 1948 offered them citizenship. Migration intensified during the 1960s and 1970s especially among those who could afford to leave. Ahmad (2005, p. 43) refers to the "push" and "pull" factors that lead to migration. One "push" factor that may explain the exodus is the race riots that took place between the African and Indian Guyanese during the 1960s (Trotz 2006). The "pull" factors may have been related to personal reasons, such as professional development and greater economic opportunities.

DOI: 10.4324/9781003269915-3

Most Guyanese women who migrated to the UK entered nursing (Beishon et al. 1995), teaching, secretarial work, or became students (Roopnarine 2013). Guyana's educational system was modelled on the British System, with English as the first language thus providing ideal entry qualifications for study or employment.

Guyana was under colonial rule at the time the study group migrated to the UK. I had not personally fully appreciated the effects of colonialism or post-colonialism on the individual or the impact it has on an individual's identity. I became enlightened by reading the literature of post-colonialist theorists such as Said (1978) and Spivak (1990) which contributed to my understanding of the post-colonial period. It is important to disentangle what happens to an individual when they migrate from a former colony to the 'mother country', and the impact this has. The effects of colonialism do not cease because of what happened in the past but continue to affect people in various ways, for example in terms of national identity. Macleod and Bhatia (2007) argue that all post-colonial societies are still subject in one way or another to subtle and hidden forms of colonial domination.

One way to resist this domination is to develop a national identity. I particularly liked the seminal work of Childs and Williams (1996) that suggests it is difficult to shed the colonial identity and develop a national identity after colonial rule. They suggest individuals ask questions such as "who are we?" when trying to develop an identity, the formation of which should be encouraged either by writing or telling one's history. Telling one's story is similar in some respects to telling one's history because it begins with a story of self that includes expressing feelings of national pride and identity (Childs & Williams 1996). PAR concurred with my belief in storytelling as a vehicle for communication. I was aware that Guyanese people liked telling stories so felt this approach would suit them to tell their stories of living with Type 2 Diabetes and feel fully involved in collaborating and creating realistic and culturally sensitive knowledge.

The eight women who volunteered for the study had been living in London an average of 40 years but did not know each other. They shared the problem of suffering from long-term diabetes. The concentration of BAME has been explained by 'choice' and 'constraint' theories (Lakey 1997). Choice theory argues that ethnic minorities prefer to live within their own group for social support and shared linguistic, cultural, and religious traditions. Constraint theory argues that ethnic minority groups are prevented from moving outside certain geographical areas by their economic position, limited knowledge of housing opportunities and fear of discrimination. Rich (1986) considered the difficulties due to racism and other prejudices affecting settlers from the West Indies who came to England from 1945 to 1962; and results in a high concentration of BAME communities in specific areas of London.

The study

I designed and submitted a PhD study proposal to the University's Ethics Committee that was approved. A poster was circulated amongst the Guyanese community and organisations in the London area. Self-selecting volunteers were sent a letter, information sheet and consent form to comply with ethics approval. My conversations with the women started in 2010. The group's questions snowballed about genetic predisposition, limited access to diabetic services and the Guyanese diet.

The selected women had a median age of 69, were middle class, well-educated and had been employed as administrators, midwives, and business partners. They had been living with diabetes for several years but were either totally unaware that they had the condition or encountered problems obtaining a diagnosis.

The philosophical underpinning for my research was based on the work of Habermas (1972, 1984) and his theoretical thinking focused on emancipation, and, like Friere (1970), Habermas's social theory advanced the goals of human participation, communicative action and dialogue as individuals meet in conversation. Habermas (1984) argued for the democratisation of research and encouraged those excluded from the process to have a voice. Consistent with Habermas's worldview is that PAR is motivated by a desire to secure authentic information (new knowledge) about people and situations that embraces experience as a source of legitimate knowledge.

Diabetes

Over 4.9 million people in the UK have diabetes (Diabetes UK 2021) now and often do not perceive they have a serious problem. Symptoms such as thirst, tiredness and frequency of micturition build up gradually. This means that at diagnosis, 20% already show signs of damage to the microvascular system, kidneys, and their sight. There is also a higher risk of heart attacks and nervous system damage leading to injury, infection, and limb loss (Watkins et al. 2003).

South Asian and African Caribbean people are respectively six and three times more likely to have Type 2 diabetes (Oldroyd et al 2005) than the white population within the UK. Cardiovascular disease, retinopathy and increased mortality are also higher among BAME groups.

Development of diabetic services

Diabetic services evolved from a pre-1970s medical model of provision where the hospital consultant assumed responsibility for the individual's care rather than the general practitioner (GP). Post-1970s, primary and community health care professionals assumed responsibility for the routine review, monitoring and management of individuals with diabetes. However, with the advent of the UK

GP contract in 1990 and payment for chronic disease management in primary care in 1993, this brought a change in focus for diabetes care (Kirby 2002) leading to care being delivered by the GP and the primary health care team (PCT).

The National Service Framework (NSF) (DH 2001) produced the first set of national standards advocating a partnership approach to care for those with Type 2 Diabetes. This framework required the health care professional and the individual to work together with the emphasis on collaborative care. National Institute and Clinical Excellence (NICE 2003) also published further standards that all individuals with diabetes should be offered structured education tailored to meet their needs, accessible across different cultures and geographical areas. In addition to the standards advocated by NICE, other self-management approaches for example the Expert Patient programme for those with diabetes were offered that included the principles of empowerment using a partnership approach. Whilst these developments were presented as significant changes to diabetic services, issues like poverty, disparity of access, and cultural barriers remained unchallenged. These developments did not seem to translate into practice for engaging BAME communities (Stone et al. 2006).

Most people with Type 2 Diabetes were treated by the GP and PCT (BMA 2012). The team agreed the practice guidelines for the management of diabetes and the roles of each member. The integrated care pathway was the preferred model clearly identifying that the individual was likely to need a variety of services during their lifetime (Young 2010).

Despite NHS improvements in diabetes care delivery there were gaps in BAME provision resulting from interventions being designed to meet the needs of a homogeneous White middle class society. Changes in legislation and policy expected health services to address inequalities (Marmot 2013; Bircher & Kuruvilla 2014) but did not do so for marginalised groups. Recognising and identifying structural factors such as health/social care policies and health care practices that maintain inequality needs to be addressed as diabetes does not affect everyone equally.

Inequalities exist in access to diabetes care and treatment. For example: Data from 2020 shows major inequalities in the number of people accessing the eight care processes that help to monitor diabetes and detect complications at an early stage. Missing out on these vital checks could mean complications go undetected and people miss out on the treatment they need. There was a 17.7% difference in the number of people accessing all eight care processes between people from ethnic minorities compared to those of White ethnicity (DH 2021).

Methodology

The PAR approach used methods of data generation consisting of storytelling interviews, focus groups and a research journal. The PAR approach endorses the centrality of storytelling in health care to transform peoples' lives.

Participants bring their own knowledge and reflection to the research process. Constant validation of this knowledge is the cornerstone of the PAR process (Koch & Kralik 2006; Koch 2015). For the researcher, keeping a journal was important because it entailed reflexivity, aided reflection, and encouraged me, as the researcher, to think about my reactions to the participants and record my feelings (Waterman 2013).

It is distinctive as a research methodology due to its focus on collaboration, political engagement, and explicit commitment to social justice (Brydon-Miller et al. 2015). Distinctive features tend to be community based and driven. Its sole purpose is to generate knowledge or understanding that leads to reform and bring about change (Baum et al. 2006; De Chesnay 2014; Bradbury 2015).

Relationship building is central to the process and participants set the agenda and take action to bring about personal change in their lives. In practical terms PAR methodology is carried out as a series of planning, acting, observing, and evaluating cycles. It allows change to evolve incrementally and be embedded into social systems. See Figure 3.1.

A particular strength in using PAR is that it is based on Paulo Friere's (1970) conscious-raising and critical awareness through practice and participation leading to community-based interventions. Friere's critical emancipatory research demonstrates that working collaboratively alongside people enables them to develop a new awareness of self which can then respond to change (Friere 1970). PAR also helps restore people's capacities of self-reliance and managing their own lives and aims to solve real problems in marginalised communities. It has been used with many groups living with a chronic illness.

The challenge of PAR is to ensure participants collaborate fully and drive the process, while acknowledging that change may not always be possible and potential power imbalances must be discussed (Gaventa & Cornwall 2015).

We[1] asked the women to tell their story about living with diabetes and the impact this has had (or not) on their lives.

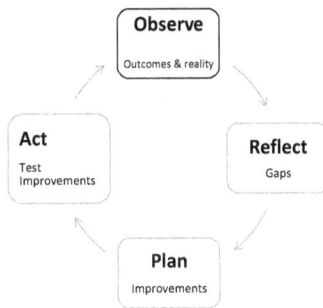

Figure 3.1 Participatory action research cycle

The researcher asked three questions:

1 What is happening in this story?
2 What has the participant chosen to talk about?
3 What is important here?'

Storytelling interviews

Guyanese people derive great benefit from telling stories, using familiar methods such as oral storytelling or pictures, guided by their memories, future hopes, and aspirations (Holloway & Freshwater 2007).

Storytelling within PAR enabled the women to act as co-researchers and to systematically resolve specific problems and decide on actions (Koch & Kralik 2006; Koch 2015). In addition, researchers listening to the stories gained understanding of the changes that the women wished to make in their daily lives (Frank 1997).

The women wanted to talk with researchers about their chronic condition. The first conversation took place in their own homes, often with two of the researchers present. Interviews were recorded and transcribed, and transcripts were returned to the women for their validation, reflection, and comment. Once we had met all the women and initial interviews were completed, we invited them to join a group.

Participatory action research groups

Group sessions were held in rotation at individual women's houses, and it was made clear that they would set the agenda for discussion. These were social events, initially with elaborate Guyanese food preparations, which became more restrained as the topic of healthy eating was placed on the group's agenda. I facilitated the group, inviting those who were elsewhere to Skype in.

We used diabetes journals, internet searches, and invited a Diabetes Specialist Nurse to two of the sessions where many questions were asked about the use of alternative herbal therapies, healthy eating, and blood sugar measurements. Listening and supporting each other were crucial actions. In each session they reported to each other what had been achieved: exercise, diet review for healthy eating, and blood testing. They became more assertive in demanding health checks but recognised how racism and discriminatory practices had delayed diagnosis and affected their relationships within the health care system.

The women's learning accelerated in the group sessions as they became more reflective or dwelled longer in the 'thinking' phase of the process. The Kolb (1984) learning cycle acted as a focus for action and evaluation of learning.

Analysis of data

The '*look, think* and *act* PAR analysis approach (Koch and Kralik 2006) was adapted to analyse the storytelling, written data, and other data collected during the PAR group sessions including reflections from participants and researcher/facilitators in the groups. *Look* consisted of a description of their story and *think* what is being reflected on. The learning process can be observed in what people do, how people interact with the world and with others, what people mean, what they value and the language which people use to describe their world. As the story continued the participant may (or may not) decide on some actions to take which is the acting phase. The researcher monitored the actions created within the action phase of the cycle. The story telling goes on and on 'in cycles' until both parties are satisfied with the 'end' product. The outcomes of these cycles are often personal growth and development for both the researcher and women. The same cycles applied to the group process. The stories were analysed, and observations provided to the women as feedback. These steps are rarely linear, so we invited the participants to reflect on the feedback and continue their stories in subsequent sessions. The journal data constituted what was going on whilst researching as self-awareness developed. Reflection in PAR is crucial for both the researcher and the participants as they rethink their position, discover new ways of being, acting and doing, and deal with the issues that they face during the research process. Schon (1983) model of reflection guided the reflection.

We honour the women's storytelling words here in the excerpts below. Names are self-selected and fictional.

Excerpts from the women's stories

Vera

I was diagnosed with diabetes but had been experiencing symptoms for 18 months. Prior to diagnosis I had experienced many symptoms and reported these to my (GP), but no tests were done. In the end it was one of my staff at work that picked up on my condition. She had been a diabetic for a long time. Then I had month's wait before an appointment to hospital for tests. I was then diagnosed with Type 2 diabetes. I monitored my medications and noticed that tablets combined with the diet were not working. I reported this to the GP and was started on insulin. Then my eyes started to give me trouble. When medical staff looked at my eyes, they talked between themselves, not to me but over my head. Without explanation they 'lasered' my eyes. I said to my family 'this cannot be right'. I saw somebody privately and when he looked at my eyes he said that I could go blind at any minute! To date my medical management has been haphazard.

Marjorie

My diabetes was first diagnosed at Easter. For about six months, I thought I had this thing because I would drink a two-litre bottle of coke in half a day. When I first noticed something was wrong, I was just getting fatter. I ate all the Guyanese food, crisps, and biscuits. I was at work on Holy Thursday that year and suddenly I went blind. I shouted to my boss Paul: "Paul I can't see!" He called a cab and phoned the doctors to make an emergency appointment. I was shocked with this diagnosis of diabetes. The doctor gave me a prescription of Metformin. I was under a medical team at a diabetic clinic at a major local hospital for a while. Then I was warned: "if you are not good at controlling your diabetes, you might have to inject insulin". Didn't get the support I needed.

Pam

Getting diabetes was something extra that came along as I already self-managed fibromyalgia and arthritis. I manage my diabetes with assistance from the diabetic nurse with whom I meet every six weeks. Before the diagnosis, my blood pressure was high, but I did not want to take any more tablets, so I said to the nurse "I'll bring it down". I regularly check my glucose levels with testers. But coming back to the diabetes, I'm not really worried about it because my mother had it when she was in her fifties, and she always managed it with diet. She lived with it for a very long time. Six of my sisters have diabetes. I'm a Buddhist and we have a great faith that the body can heal itself. I try to have a lot of leafy green vegetables and water-based fruit because that is what the body needs, more water. I know I can take care of myself.

Bea

My diabetes was first diagnosed twenty years ago. I come from a family of known diabetics. One of the first symptoms was that I felt dizzy. It was totally out of the blue one day that the GP told me to come to the surgery and I had the fasting glucose test done. Only then did he inform me that I was diabetic. Yes, sometimes people do exhibit symptoms such as feeling very thirsty, but I can't remember feeling like that. Once diagnosed I self-managed with diet. Later I took a drug called metformin. Then there was a problem with my kidneys. Eventually my GP took heed and had me investigated. I am now on insulin. I worry about my family getting diabetes. I know I have a family history and how little had been understood or done for my mother and father.

Jane

I was diagnosed with diabetes about ten years ago after I retired from my position at a department store. I did not have any symptoms but was aware that my father and grandparents had died from this condition, so I took preventive action by checking regularly from the day I came to England to see if I had acquired it. It took a while to be diagnosed and I was on a diet only for the first three years and then tablets. During the early stages of the condition, my glucose levels were perfect in the daytime but when I went to sleep and woke up in the mornings, my sugar levels were always high and that is the case up to now. I was sweating a lot during the night because I hadn't eaten all night and the consultant believed that I was having a hypoglycaemic coma. The consultant suggested that I eat a slice of bread before going to bed and the sweating eventually stopped. About two years ago I was started on insulin. I take insulin once a day at night.

Shirley

When I was diagnosed, I just wasn't feeling right. I saw the doctor several times, but she didn't know what was wrong. She put it down to stress. In the end I was diagnosed with diabetes. I have been on tablets since then, Metformin, which I am on now. I had to change my eating habits, as I never liked to eat regularly. I ate erratically, so I had to eat at the correct time. Coming back to the management of diabetes and food, I never liked sweet things. Sweet things do not have anything to do with diabetes, it is another myth, but Guyanese eat a lot of sugary foods. I don't like cooking. Someone said you can't come from Guyana and don't like to cook. I said: 'I am sure not all Guyanese like cooking'.

Agnes

The reason for coming to England was to join my husband. I retired nearly four years ago from the Housing Benefit office. Before I was diagnosed with diabetes, I noticed that I had a problem when I got up in the morning. I would feel dizzy and have blurred vision, so I decided to make an appointment with the GP. I was prescribed Metformin and asked to attend diabetic classes. I have been going regularly to the clinic, where they test my blood sugar to see if the level has increased. My husband and son used herbal remedies to treat their diabetes. I just use the medication. My husband had a stroke and passed away. We had a coroner's inquest that brought some closure, but when I came home that afternoon after the hearing, I almost fainted. My son said: 'mum you need to go and rest'. I was admitted to hospital about three weeks ago. I heard them saying that I had a problem with my heart.

Jillian

I was diagnosed with Type 2 diabetes following a visit to my husband's brother in Guyana. His wife noticed that I was losing weight. He who is also a diabetic, gave me a blood test using his equipment. My blood sugar reading was 14. It had not occurred to me that I had diabetes as I did not have the usual symptoms like being thirsty or anything like that. But I have a family history of diabetes. Both of my parents were diabetic. My mother died from kidney failure. She used to be on insulin, but my father lived to a good old age. I have a sister (a nun) who is diabetic, and my daughter was diagnosed at university when she was in her early twenties.

We arrived in England in November 1964, and it was so cold. We had been married for many years when he died from dementia. When he became ill, I used to give him his insulin because he had diabetes too.

Discussion

Diagnosis of Type 2 diabetes

Delay in being diagnosed was not uncommon for some women before they received a confirmed diagnosis as observed in their stories. Some had experienced a fragmented, inconsistent, and non-responsive service delivery model with dire consequences for their health. They were experiencing symptoms of Type 2 Diabetes such as dizziness, extreme thirst, blurred vision, feeling tired, drinking copious amounts of fluids and weight loss (DH 2010) yet these warning signs did not alert health care practitioners that something was wrong. It required the women to be assertive with the health care providers about their need for care and attention e.g., tests, testing equipment, request for tablets and/or insulin. It seemed that their voices were not heard.

Receiving a diagnosis from the GP confirmed an acceptance that the individual is genuinely ill and encompassed an explanation for their symptoms of diabetes (Richardson et al. 2001; Parry et al. 2004). People react differently when a diagnosis has been confirmed. This reaction has been likened to bereavement where the individual can go through a period of disbelief, anger, shock, and denial (Peel et al. 2004). Marjorie stated in her story that she was shocked when she received the initial diagnosis but then realised "you learn to live with it". Jillian who was unaware of what was happening to her, sought help from her GP after a relative with diabetes observed her weight loss, tested her glucose levels, and highlighted it was raised. Research by Koopman et al. (2004) revealed that people are unaware of the meaning of their symptoms of diabetes even though they may be exhibiting them because the symptoms appear to be vague. Individuals may also choose to ignore their symptoms due to fear that can act as a barrier when seeking consultation with their GP rather than acknowledge that they have a condition like Type 2 Diabetes (Koopman et al. 2004). Surprisingly some of the women were still shocked that they had Type 2 Diabetes even with a known family history and regular visits to the GP.

Doctor-patient relationship

Dissatisfaction with the doctor-patient relationship was a reoccurring theme in the women's stories. They shared with me the communication problems that existed between them and their GPs following diagnosis. Miscommunication and feeling ignored were key issues in the doctor-patient relationship which May et al. (2004) state is not new, particularly in the consultations where there may be disagreement regarding what was said. This disagreement is normally attributed to poor recall when decisions are made between the two parties (Parkin & Skinner 2003). There is also the assumption that the doctor knows best and is the expert rather than developing a relationship with the individual based on mutual respect. The women found this a challenge as they tried to navigate their way through the diabetic services and to engage in a meaningful relationship with their respective GPs. They preferred to be seen as an individual with specific needs rather than as 'a patient'.

Racism

The women had experienced a reversal of class when they migrated to the UK and for the first time experienced being from a BAME community. I am particularly aware of the struggles some of them faced when they came in the 1950s and 1960s especially Bea and Vera who spoke openly about their experiences in the group sessions. As Bea said, "One notice on the door said coloured people and dogs were not welcome". Others found it difficult to cope with life in the UK even though they had acquired very responsible positions. Vera talked about the problems she encountered at work and said, "I could have put my coat on and walked out and never looked back, but I kept at it".

Bea discussed the racism that she faced as a midwife but said that she and her friend were trail blazers in midwifery as they were the first 'coloured' midwives to visit English people in their homes to deliver babies. They felt it was important to know your place in the social structure and the difficulties experienced if you tried to move away from that structure. Back (2005) postulates that racism is normally defined as a form of spatial and territorial form of power that aims to secure a particular territory which the other claim as their own. Back (2005) claims people develop a map of belonging to make that territory their home even though risks are involved as they cross boundaries. Being 'Black' in a white society signifies only 'whiteness' according to (Alleyne 2002) as Black people aim to seek recognition of their value and dignity and oppose racial stereotypes. These women had to learn how to transcend racism in those early days and realised their identity was strong as they shared experiences and spoke with pride about their home country and what it was like to be Guyanese. They developed profound loyalty and found support from each other. They had left Guyana years ago but retained their identity as they grappled with oppression and marginalisation. The experiences of discrimination and race had re-emerged as they tried to obtain a diagnosis for diabetes.

We pondered whether it is more likely that women of colour are not heard in the NHS system? Women talked about racism and discrimination in one-to-one conversations but did not want to pursue this as a group. Szczepura (2005) reviewed the research evidence on access to health care by ethnic minority populations and highlighted that it has not been possible to develop a UK overview of disparities in access to the service because the data do not provide sufficiently detailed information. She believed that

> simply providing an equal service cannot ensure access to care for all people, regardless of their religion, culture, or ethnic background. Having access to services should be relevant, timely and sensitive to the person's needs with confidence that you will be treated with respect.
>
> (Szczepura 2005: 142)

Bea said in her story and group sessions that she made every effort to access the GP by contacting him regularly, yet it took a long time before the condition was diagnosed even with a family history.

The women identified the kind of diabetic service that was preferable, one that was consultative with a holistic approach to the care and treatment. They believed the "one size fits all model" currently provided for all individuals with Type 2 diabetes was not culturally appropriate for those with specific beliefs and needs because it did not address cultural variations, underlying motivations, preferences, and behaviours.

Reflection

Throughout this journey, I maintained a reflective journal. I queried if and how my role as a woman/researcher/facilitator/registered nurse/Guyanese expatriate/UK citizen was influencing and/or working as a change agent. My critical stance shifted noticeably. For instance, I initially took for granted my Guyanese background and identity. I did not at first see the way in which women embraced each other culturally to learn collaboratively. It took my PhD supervisors to point out how exceptional that was. I'd say it took a few years of critical reflection before I was able to see that all my identities had impacted on the study. I reignited one of those identities in finding myself to be proudly Guyanese. Arriving in the UK, and living an English life, this was also an opportunity to reconnect with London's Guyanese community. I am now motivated to instigate further Guyanese group studies in the UK and in Guyana.

Conclusion

In this inquiry we have heard the women's voices about living with Type 2 diabetes. Women expressed a strong sense of self-development and evolution in their lives, they demonstrated an increased understanding of their situation, and the group-initiated action. My task was to provide the women with the support and resources to do things in their own way. The women decided on the nature of things that affected their lives: they set the agenda. I claim that bringing these women together enhanced their diabetes self-management. Questioning self-management was accelerated within the PAR group. The women questioned their food choices often, recognising that 'traditional foods could not be construed as healthy eating: healthy eating is a prerequisite for diabetes self-management. The inquiry came to an end, but self-management of a chronic condition is a lifelong learning process. Sustainability is a success indicator for PAR. In this way, it is not surprising that women were still learning but that bringing them together as a group accelerated learning and improvements in their health.

Note

1 Although I led the research, my two supervisors were present at some of the individual interviews and PAR group meetings.

References

Ahmad, O. B. (2005) Managing medical migration from poor countries. *British Medical Journal*. **331** (7507), pp. 43–45.

Alleyne M. C. (2002) *The Construction and Representation of Race and Ethnicity in the Caribbean and the World*. University of the West Indies Press, Jamaica.

Back L. (2005) 'Home from home': youth, belonging and place. In Alexander C. & Knowles C. (eds.) *Making Race Matter: Bodies, Space & Identity*. Palgrave, Basingstoke, pp. 19–41.

Baum F., MacDougall C., & Smith D. (2006) Participatory action research. *Journal of Epidemiology Community Health*. **60** (10), pp. 854–857.

Beishon S., Satnam V., & Hagell A. (1995) *Nursing in a Multi-ethnic NHS*. Policy Studies Institute, London.

Bircher, J. & Kuruvilla, S. (2014) Defining health by addressing individual, social, and environmental determinants: new opportunities for health care and public health. *Journal of Public Health Policy*. **35** (3), pp. 363–86. doi: 10.1057/jphp.2014.19

Bradbury H., ed. (2015) *The Handbook of Action Research*. Sage, London.

British Medical Association (BMA) (2012) *Quality and Outcomes Framework 2012/2013 – Guidance for PCOs and Practices*. (Online). Available from: bma.org.uk/-/media/Files/Pdfs/Practical (Accessed 15 July 2013).

Brydon-Miller M., Aranda A. R., & Stevens D. M. (2015) Widening the circle: ethical reflection in action research and the practice of structured ethical reflection. In Bradbury H. (ed.) *The Handbook of Action Research*. Sage, London, pp. 596–607.

Childs P. & Patrick Williams R. J. (1996) *An Introduction to Post-Colonial Theory*. Prentice Hall, London.

De Chesnay M. (2014) *Nursing Research Using Participatory Action Research: Qualitative Designs and Methods in Nursing*. New York, Springer Publishing Company.

Department of Health (2001) *National Service Frameworks for Diabetes: Standards*. Department of Health, London.

Department of Health (2010) *Six years On: Delivering the Diabetes National Service Framework*. Department of Health, London.

Department of Health (2021) Health and Care Bill. https://publications.parliament.uk/pa/cm5802/cmpublic/HealthCare/memo/HCB20.htm. Accessed 12.1.2023.

Frank A. W. (1997) *The Wounded Storyteller.* The University of Chicago Press, London.

Friere P. (1970) *Pedagogy of the Oppressed.* Continuum, New York.

Gaventa, J., Cornwall, A. (2015) Power and knowledge. In Bradbury, H. (ed.) *The Sage handbook of action research: Participative inquiry and practice* (3rd ed.). Sage, Thousand Oaks, CA, pp. 465–471.

Green S. M., & Emanuel S. (2000) *Social Studies Guyana.* Caribbean Educational Publishers, Trinidad.

Habermas J. (1972) *Knowledge and Human Interests.* Heinemann, London.

Habermas J. (1984) *The Theory of Communicative Action. Vol 2: Lifeworld and System: A critique of Functionalist Reason.* Beacon Press, Boston, MA.

Holloway I., & Freshwater D. (2007) Vulnerable story telling: narrative research in nursing. *Journal of Research in Nursing.* **12** (6), pp. 703–711.

Kirby M. (2002) Fifty years of diabetes management in primary care. *British Journal of Diabetes and Vascular Disease.* **2** (6), pp. 457–461.

Koch T. (2015) Improving health and well being: researching alongside marginalised people across diverse domains. In Bradbury H. (ed.) *The Sage Handbook of Action Research* (3rd ed.). Sage, London, pp. 325–335.

Koch T., & Kralik D. (2006) *Participatory Action Research in Health Care.* Blackwell, Carlton.

Kolb D. A. (1984) *Experiential Learning: Experience as the Source of Learning and Development.* Prentice-Hall, New York.

Koopman R. J., Manous A. G. & Jeffcoat A. S. (2004) Moving from undiagnosed to diagnosed diabetes: the patient's perspective. *Family Medicine.* **36** (10), pp. 727–732.

Lakey J. (1997) Neighbourhoods and housing. In Modood T., Berthoud R., Lakey J., Nazroo J., Smith P., Virdee S. & Beishon S. (eds.) *Ethnic Minorities in Britain: Diversity and Disadvantage. Fourth National survey of Ethnic Minorities.* Policy Studies Institute, London, pp. 184–223.

Macleod C., & Bhatia S. (2007) Post colonialism and psychology. In Willig C. & Stainton-Rogers W. (eds.) *The Sage Handbook of Qualitative Research in Psychology.* Sage, London, pp. 576–589.

Marmot, M. (2013) WHO European Review. Available at: https://www.instituteofhealthequity.org/projects/who-european-review

May C., Allison G., Chapple A., Chew-Grahan C., Dixon C., Gask L., Graham R., Rogers A., & Roland M. (2004) Framing the doctor-patient relationship in chronic illness: a comparative study of general practitioners' accounts. *Sociology of Health and Illness.* **26** (2), pp. 135–158.

National Institute for Clinical Excellence (NICE) (2003) The clinical effectiveness and cost effectiveness of patient education models for diabetes (online). Available from: www.nice.org.uk/guidance/index.sp?action=byIDxr (Accessed 30 July 2012).

National Institute for Health and Clinical Excellence (NICE) (2009) Type 2 Diabetes (online). Available from: www.nice.org.uk/nicemedia/live/12165/44322/44322.pdf (Accessed 10 April 2013).

Oldroyd J., Banerjee M., Heald A., & Cruickshank K. (2005) Diabetes and ethnic minorities. *Postgraduate Medical Journal.* **81** (958), pp. 486–490.

Parkin T., & Skinner T. C. (2003) Discrepancies between patient and professionals recall and perception of an outpatient consultation. *Diabetic Medicine.* **20** (1), pp. 909–914.

Parry O., Peel E., Douglas M., & Lawton J. (2004) Patients in waiting: a qualitative study of type 2 diabetes patients' perceptions of diagnosis. *Family Practice.* **21**, pp. 131–136.

Peel E., Parry O., Douglas M., & Lawton J. (2004) Diagnosis of type 2 diabetes: a qualitative analysis of patients' emotional reactions and views about information provision. *Patient Education Counselling.* **53** (3), pp. 269–275.

Rich P. (1986) Black people in Britain. *History Today* (online). **36** (1). Available from: www.historytoday.com/paul-rich/black-people-britain-response-an (Accessed 17/1/2023).

Richardson A., Adner N., & Nordstrom G. (2001) Persons with insulin dependent mellitus: acceptance and coping ability. *Journal of Advanced Nursing.* **33** (6), pp. 758–763.

Roopnarine L. (2013) *Guyana Population Movement and Social Development.* Institute of Development Studies 50th anniversary Working Paper Series – Working Paper 7/12 (online), University of Guyana. Available from: idsguyana.org (Accessed 14 March 2014).

Said E. (1978) *Orientalism.* Penguin Books, London.

Schon D. A. (1983) *The Reflective Practitioner.* New York, Basic Books.

Spivak G. C. (1990) *The Postcolonial Critic: Interviews, Strategies, Dialogues.* Routledge, New York.

Stone M. A., Patel N., Drake L., & Gayle C. (2006) Making education in diabetes culturally appropriate for patients. *Practice Nursing.* **17** (12), pp. 621–625.

Szczepura A. (2005) Access to health care for ethnic minority populations. *Postgraduate Medical Journal.* **81** (953), pp. 141–147.

Trotz A. (2006) Rethinking Caribbean transnational connections: conceptual itineraries. *Global Networks.* **6** (1), pp. 41–59.

Waterman H. (2013) Action research and health. In Saks M. and Allsop J. (eds.) *Researching Health* (2nd ed.). Sage, London, pp. 148–167.

Watkins P. J., Amiel S. A., Howell L. S., & Turner E. (2003) *Diabetes and Its Management.* (6th ed.) Blackwell, Oxford.

Young B. (2010) The organisation of diabetes care. *Journal of Royal College Physicians.* **17** (40), pp. 33–39.

4 Experiences of perinatal British mental health services

Reflections on conducting research with migrant women from Sub-Saharan Africa

Gabriel Ngalomba

Introduction to chapter

As an African migrant healthcare professional working in perinatal mental health services (PNMHS), I was aware of what appeared to be institutional and structural racism faced by migrant Sub-Saharan African women in PNMHS. This awareness drove my eagerness to conduct research involving a group of migrant Sub-Saharan women to understand their lived experiences after using PNMHS in the UK. In this chapter, I reflect on the experience of being a PhD student who shares ethnicity with a group of research participants.

This study was conducted in the context of my witnessing global campaigns such as that of Black Lives Matter (BLM) which heightened society's perception of the oppression of people of black ethnicity while at the same time working as a nurse in the care of migrant women of Sub-Saharan African origin in PNMHS. These two experiences influenced my use of Critical Race Theory (CRT) as the theoretical framework for discussing the findings.

Perinatal Mental Health Services in the UK

PNMHS are services designed to offer support and treatment to women who suffer from mental health conditions during pregnancy to a year postnatally. These services offer both inpatient and community support to women who experience all forms of mental illness in the UK. These range from common perinatal mental health problems such as perinatal depression, anxiety, and phobia, to severe postpartum psychosis, bipolar affective disorder, and post-traumatic stress disorder (The National Institute for Health and Care Excellence (NICE), 2016).

There are 22 inpatient mother and baby units and around 40 community PNMHS in the UK. The use of services is dependent on the risk level and severity of the illness women can experience. These services are under the guidance of the Royal College of Psychiatrists, the main professional body of psychiatrists that provides public information about mental health problems (National Collaborating Centre for Mental Health et al., 2011).

DOI: 10.4324/9781003269915-4

The Royal College of Psychiatrists has recommended that inpatient admissions for pregnant women whose risks are too high to be managed in the communities, take place from 32 weeks of pregnancy up to a year postnatally (Royal College of Psychiatrists, 2018).

In its long-term plan, the Department of Health and Social Care aims to improve PNMHS for all women with symptoms irrespective of their ethnic backgrounds and ensure that are treated in specialist services (National Health Services UK, 2019). Despite the efforts from the Department of Health and Social Care and various charitable organisations to raise awareness about perinatal mental illness and available services, there is evidence that marginalised groups of women are reluctant to accept a diagnosis of mental illness (Department of Health, 2016; Smith et al., 2019).

Introduction to PhD

Working in the NHS placed me in a position to see the impact of institutional racism on the migrant women of Sub-Saharan African origin who accessed these services as most of them were unable to access services as early as their white counterparts, in other words they accessed services later than is desired. As a result, their access to PNMHS was under the Mental Health Act or Social Services orders i.e. involuntary admission. Literature suggests that black and ethnic minority women are four times more likely to be placed under a compulsory admission order in PNMHS in the United Kingdom compared to white women (NHS Digital, 2021).

Sharing culture and ethnicity with the research participants in my study allowed me to gain insights into women's experiences of institutional and structural racism in PNMHS while analysing the role of gender in our shared culture and ethnicity.

There is evidence to suggest that some migrant women, including those of Sub-Saharan African origin, are reluctant to access services due to what appears to be a fear of structural and institutional racism (Bansal et al., 2022; Pilav et al., 2022). As a result, their mental state deteriorates to the extent of reaching a crisis point. These women try to engage in other therapies in order to alleviate their challenges, which to a great extent makes their journey into PNMHS more challenging as their treatments tend to take longer due to the delayed untreated perinatal mental illness (Ling et al., 2023; Pangas et al., 2019).

Methodological framework for the PhD: Husserlian descriptive phenomenology

Since the aim of this study was to understand the Sub-Saharan African migrant women's lived experiences of British PNMHS during pregnancy and after giving birth in the past five years, I felt that using phenomenology as my methodological framework helped me to get a sense of what it was like

to be a service user and how this affected their day to day lives. Phenomenology is guided by the principle that human beings are self-reflective people
in their day-to-day lives, reflecting on their experiences in life and societies
in which they live, which can be a valuable source of data to understand
them (Giorgi, 2012). The two main traditions within phenomenology are
descriptive phenomenology by Husserl (Giorgi, 2012) and interpretive (Hei-
deggerian) phenomenology (Reiners, 2012). Husserlian phenomenology
prompts researchers to conceal their views or opinions and rely on the research participants' narratives of their lived experiences (Pitard, 2017). This
is described as bracketing or epoche. Heidegger's interpretive phenomenological approach argues that our understanding of daily life is derived from
how we perceive the world, and it is not easy to bracket our experiences and
knowledge related to a phenomenon as what we know (ontology) and how
we know (epistemology) may affect and guide what we want to enquire into
and our findings (Christensen and Lægreid, 2017).

In this study, I used descriptive phenomenology as my interest was to understand descriptions of lived experiences of migrant women of Sub-Saharan
African origin in the United Kingdom. Bracketing what I know about perinatal mental illness helped me to elicit women's lived experiences without
making assumptions or judgement when women gave their narratives during
interviews. Using this approach, I aimed to report the exact meaning as described by research participants. Bracketing my experiences with this group
of women during data collection helped because of my positioning. I have
not experienced perinatal mental illness, and being a man means that I am in
a different position to the women I interviewed: although I care as a nurse for
women in PNMHS, I have not experienced mental illness.

However, during data collection using unstructured interviews, I felt that
engaging in 'epoche', caused a clear tension between what I know about the
topic and the need to put my knowledge aside, to gather the participants' lived
experiences as I shared ethnicity with my participants. Bracketing my preconceived ideas about what I know about this group of women did not seem
to help my data collection and interpretation without altering meaning. Being
seen by women as sharing ethnicity did not change the study aims but meant
that I struggled with using the methodology as a new researcher. I retained
an awareness, a reflective stance, which made me as a researcher remain cautious not to influence any narrative as given by research participants. This
stance shaped my interview method of using unstructured interviews so that
my presence as a researcher sharing ethnicity did not influence the research
participants' narratives on their lived experiences. However, during interviews, the participants' narratives did not stop my mind from thinking about
what research participants experienced because of my shared ethnicity. This
may be one of the limitations of Husserl's descriptive phenomenology as it
was not possible to bracket and not relate to issues affecting black ethnicity.
I was able to recognise these limitations of Husserlian bracketing but this did
not stop me from eliciting the women's lived experiences while at the same

time developing my own methodology around shared positioning in research between participants and myself as a researcher. To mitigate this, I used excerpts from reflections in a research diary to illustrate the experiences of both the women and me as researcher as an additional research tool. Furthermore, constant reminders that my position was to gather their lived experiences appeared to have cemented my stance on the aim of the study. These women were made aware that my main intention was to ensure that their voices were heard. The use of direct quotes from these women is my evidence to show I reported their voices.

Theoretical framework: Critical Race Theory

Following the Sub-Saharan migrant women's lived experiences in relation to the PNMHS care they received, and after reflecting in supervision following analysis of my research diary during data analysis, I chose CRT as my theoretical framework in my discussion chapter.

This framework is centred on the argument that various institutions in western societies including health care systems are structured by racist ideology based on white supremacy which discriminate against individuals based on their colour of their skin (Adebayo et al., 2022; Huddle, 2022). In short, CRT assumes that race and racial classification are socially constructed, and people of colour have suffered marginalisation and oppression over time (See Chapter 1). However, their lived experiences or narratives can be used to bring about changes (Delgado and Stefancic, 1993). The above argument, which was echoed by the Sub-Saharan migrant women in the UK, confirmed my decision to use CRT as my theoretical framework in my research at the data analysis stage. It seemed especially pertinent as according to Delgado and Stepfacic (2023), CRT states that social institutions are racist which leads to unequal services provisions, which includes the existence of disparities in health care provisions among ethnic groups.

Looking at the route into PNMHS by the Sub-Saharan migrant women for example, the Royal College of Psychiatrists' stipulation is that all women at perinatal period should access PNMHS without being separated from their babies.[1] The PNMHS are geared to accept women from mild to severe presentation of their mental state. But for Sub-Saharan migrant women this has not always been the case as their route has been through general mental health services where their babies are temporarily removed from them. This to a great extent causes disruption and irritability due to fear of not knowing about their care and what has happened to their babies. To some extent, limited information about the existence of PNMHS and what they entail can make one experience paranoid thoughts (National Institute for Health and Care Excellence, 2014).

In theory, contacts with health services start at the first trimester of pregnancy for all women (The Royal College of Psychiatrists, 2018). However, this group of women are not made familiar with the British health care system, how to access services of which some of them have been reported to have discriminatory practices (Latif, 2014). These fears and paranoid thoughts may be due to these women's migrant status and lack of integration into British society.

Shared ethnicity, positionality, and reflexivity

Ethnicity, grouping people with common attributes such as ancestry, cultural traditions, history, language, spiritual beliefs, and social interactions (Segal, 2019), is used globally by scholars in social sciences, humanities, and health (Helberg-Proctor et al., 2017). Shared ethnicity between a researcher and researched can be a source of inspiration in generating rich data as the researcher is not only seen as an insider but also trusted as an individual who create an opportunity for research participants to feel valued and have their voices heard (Abbas, 2006; Kerstetter, 2012). Sharing ethnicity between a researcher and participants in the context of how research is conducted, intersect to influence a good environment for a robust study (Joseph et al., 2021).

Although a researcher interviewing a familiar population can experience a comfortable environment of being an insider, this may also be seen as a challenge particularly when it comes to exploring sensitive issues which can make a researcher find it difficult to tease out how participants feel being interviewed by an insider (Courture et al., 2021). In my case, the intersectionality between myself as a researcher and the Sub-Saharan migrant women meeting in the PNMHS influenced this study from recruitment to data collection process as I sought to gain trust in these women. I believe I succeeded.

My other initial instinct was that being a male researcher who, whether they shared ethnicity or not could be challenging in getting the narratives from research participants as we did not share gender. But this was not the case as the research participants had proactively shown willingness to have their voices heard. Although the Sub-Saharan migrant women are considered to be a hard-to-reach group in research participation, my sharing ethnicity gave me an advantage in working with this group of migrant women and eliciting their experiences for this study even though I was a man.

Almost all the research participants who were willing to take part in this research reported that they felt comfortable for me to interview them as they treated me as the insider despite me not been their named nurse during their time of accessing the perinatal mental health service. This was evidenced by the rapport built with these research participants in the two meetings I had with each of them during recruitment and interviews processes. Calling me "their brother" during interviews made me believe that it illustrated the trust felt by these women towards me. However, I was aware that their trust in me could also pose a risk of response Bias as participants may only give information that they believe a researcher would like to hear (Palaniappan and Kum, 2019).

The inclusion criteria of targeting those women who were already discharged, aimed to increase honest responses as these research participants had nothing to do with the PNMHS at the time of taking part in this study. This might also imply that they did not have a fear of voicing their lived experiences of the service and challenges they encountered. A detailed explanation of my research aim using the participant information sheet seemed to have helped in increasing understanding of the aim of my study and building trust. Although there was an option of using other languages during my data collection period, most of these women preferred to be interviewed in the English language which is commonly spoken in many of the Sub-Saharan African countries as most of these African countries were under British colonial rule. Also the majority of these women moved to the UK, and had to learn English in order to communicate with others in the UK. Therefore, communication was not a problem.

Reflexivity, self-awareness, and self-reference in the process of collecting data and analysis (Ahmad, 2022; Davies, 2008), helped me as a researcher to be aware of my position (Allan and Arber, 2018) and reduced any risk of influencing findings which would have been caused by sharing ethnicity. Although four themes were identified in my findings, I am only going to discuss one theme on racism following insights gained from having shared an ethnicity in the process of research.

The findings on racism

A key finding was that most of the women I interviewed had experienced racism when using British health care services in general and PNMHS in particular. These experiences were shaped by their positioning within British society and in particular their migration status and ethnicity.

> It happens, sometimes when you are in a mental health institution people will discriminate you a little bit- I am a human being, and I did not choose to be black.
>
> (p. 11)

During interviews, it appeared that those participants who assumed a better social status, or legal immigration status or those who had been in the UK longer, did not openly report racism at both institutional and individual levels. One of the reasons might be due to various obstacles they experienced before entering or settling in the UK. Such challenges may have compelled them to learn to cope with whatever difficulties they encountered in their day-to-day dealings and racism is one of those challenges. This was evidenced by seven research participants who were cautious to talk about racism but understood that their lived experiences when in contact with the UK healthcare system could be described as racism. The narratives from research participants 1 and

2 demonstrate this. Participant 1 who had severe postpartum psychosis with her first child, was not considered for PNMHS with her second pregnancy as she was allowed to go home despite the raised concerns around high risk of relapse of her illness. But participant 1 did not see her experiences were a result of institutional racist service which goes against the Department of Health's long-term plan of supporting high-risk women to access PNMHS immediately.

> There is no like racism or anything in perinatal mental health services.
>
> (p. 1)

However, this statement seemed to change as the interview progressed and the participant described what appeared to be as a result of structural or in-stitutional racism, as despite being at high risk of relapse of her mental state, professionals did not act on time to reduce any risk.

> Some of us with mental health issues relapse due to pressure on de-livery…. may be before or after delivery I should have straight away been taken in a mother and baby unit… I should not have been left to relapse…. I wouldn't have relapsed.
>
> (p. 1)

That research participants from better socio-economic backgrounds do not openly talk about racism but internalise their experiences instead is echoed by Karisen and Nazroo (2002). Participant 2 who reported having a stable ca-reer and ability to access both UK and African health care services, reported what appeared to be an act of institutional racism when she migrated to the UK in the 20th week of her pregnancy, and transferred her obstetric care to the UK's health care services. But participant 2 was cautious to confirm this despite being told by a health care professional that some medication does not work for black people. Yet there was not any suggestion on alternative medication that could treat her condition.

> I had traumatic birth…my blood pressure was so high. so, one nurse said some of the BP medication they do not work for black people. I felt like they did not really care and wanted me to go home. no assessment was done on me…. if they treated my blood pressure, I would not get to the stage I got… I have a history of Blood pressure in family.
>
> (p. 2)

Although the World Health Organisation (2017) calls for comprehensive physical checks for migrant women at perinatal periods, this appeared to be lacking. Professionals' lack of interest and urgency to understand the women's challenges and vulnerability could be seen as another example to demonstrate the existence of institutional racist behaviour. Despite the child-bearing Sub-Saharan African migrant women's high risk of adverse maternal outcomes, there is evidence of delay in identifying their needs during a peri-natal period (Binder et al., 2012).

> But when I was telling them I was having headaches and they would say it is okay nothing is serious. Probably if I was back home in Africa, they would have known what medication that would work for me.
>
> (p. 2)

Another participant who disclosed that she came to the UK as an illegal im-migrant, reported facing racism at an individual level when accessing the perinatal mental health service:

> The white girls ganged against me because I didn't do anything to them and the way they said she is black, and they did think they are going to bring a white They were just racist, and they made things worse for me.
>
> (p. 3)

Although some migrant women might have not been affected by any act of racism at an individual level, it appeared that institutional racism could be faced by any individual irrespective of her social or immigration status. The use of Mental Health Act powers without thorough assessment for capacity can be used as an example to demonstrate this argument.

> They were going to section me without any thorough assessment as they claimed that I did not have capacity. But I really had the capacity.
>
> (p. 2)

As mentioned before, black ethnic minority individuals are four times more likely to be placed under compulsory admission order to access PNMHS in the United Kingdom (NHS Digital, 2021). Participant 10 and four argued explicitly that the decisions about their care were made without their involve-ment and in many instances, they were not given time for assessment.

> The report written about my mental health was wrong. But was not even given the opportunity to correct in their reports. So, all wrong information.
>
> (p. 10)

> I think a lot needs to be done when it comes to black Africans in our health and mental health issues not to assume. Before they brought me to Mother and baby unit, they were even planning to section me.
>
> (p. 4)

This to a great extent led to the decision about their care being made on an assumption basis as the health care professionals did not give time for explanation and assessment to take place and come up with a collaborative care plan which would be effective for these women.

> There was a lady doing one to one with me, they didn't leave me. When I am sleeping somebody was there, like I'm going outside somebody was there following me. I was like what's going on because did not have any information.
>
> (p. 3)

There was also evidence to suggest that some migrant women of Sub-Saharan African origin were reluctant to access the services due to fear of racism. As the result, their mental state deteriorated to the extent of reaching a crisis point. Some migrant women reported that they were on strong doses of medication and were not given any information about medication that they were given. As the result, they had severe side effects.

> ... I was on a high dose of medication, and I was like someone who drunk alcohol.
>
> (p. 5)

These experiences confirmed the anxiety shared in their respective communities which lead to reluctance to access services on a voluntary basis (Bansal et al., 2022; Pilav et al., 2022). For example, some research participants believed that PNMHS were associated with aggressive treatments which may lead to permanent dependency on the services.

> I found it stressful, and I was nervous. Because you are incapable. If I was sectioned, I would not have recovered as I have now as they would be there giving you injections just like that.
>
> (p. 2)

Similarly, some women narrated that they were not given options of talking therapy or any other therapeutic activities which they attributed this to their colour of their skin. But the same option was offered to white service users. When they questioned this, they were included in therapeutic groups.

> I was the only black lady, all were white I could still see the difference as there was a group, I was surprised only until I spoke when next time I was called. I didn't think I belonged there.
>
> (p. 10)

These women also reported that their physical health was not attended to, despite them making frequent visits to Maternity and Accident and Emergency departments. Instead, they were asked to return home. For example, one woman, who had pre-eclampsia did not receive the appropriate treatment until she reached a severe crisis point needing emergency C-section as failure to do so would lead to the mother and baby death. There is evidence to suggest that medical conditions such as pre-eclampsia, physical discomfort, insomnia, birth related trauma and infection can cause psychological impact in women at postpartum periods which can be triggers for postpartum mental illness (Bergink et al., 2015). All participants reported some form of discomfort which played part in their mental health deterioration.

> The doctor came to speak to me that I had preeclampsia. They were giving me antibiotics. My placenta had ruptured. My son was also on antibiotics because he was almost losing his life, he was not breathing properly so they had to take him to the intensive care unit, and they took me to a recovery Ward and put a lot of machines.
>
> (Participant 2)

Other women reported that poor sleep and abnormal blood results may have contributed to this as their appetite was also poor:

> "they took my blood sample and they said look at your sugar is down your blood is down, So, you need medical attention"
>
> (p. 3).

All these experiences indicate poor practice which contradicts the World Health Organisation (2018) guidance which reiterates the importance of getting a comprehensive medical history of migrant women during the perinatal period as part of prevention. This was not the case for most of the research participants.

Similarly, one woman described despite making frequent visits to the hospital, the professionals left her problems untreated until she reached a life-threatening point:

> The doctor only said that I had pre-eclampsia, but I was not on any medication. I was asking myself so the monitor and everything isn't that the midwife did not see what was going on and she was coming to induce me and what if the doctor had not walked in what would have happened?
>
> (p. 2)

Similarly, there was a delay in the diagnosis of perinatal mental illness and accessing the service. This according to these women was known to those health care professionals. But there was no urgency in looking for measures to treat the problem.

Being given a wrong diagnosis without culture awareness during assessment is another example of institutional racism. This was mainly associated with the research participants' cultural or spiritual beliefs which oblige them to perform certain rituals which in western society appears to be categorised as mental illness. For example, most of the research participants reported being religious and praying as one of their coping strategies which they learned from their ancestors. But for them, they reported that their spiritual beliefs made them to be treated differently. From this perspective, it appears that the clash in beliefs between the Sub-Saharan migrant women and health care professionals was caused by the latter's lack of interest in understanding cultural beliefs.

> I would say it is because of my faith which came about. I have been born and then brought up in a Christian family as my father was a pastor and my mom was reverent, I was caught up in the bubble and it brought up a lot of confusion that's why I ended up in the mental health team.
>
> (p. 4)

This emanated from professionals' lack of time to do thorough assessments to understand the migrant women's needs. For these women, not being understood as one of the barriers which they reported to have also contributed to their reluctance in accessing PNMHS.

Some women attempted to express their preferences to have their needs understood, but professionals did not give them an opportunity to be listened to. This may be due to the professionals' preconceived ideas about the Sub-Saharan African women's culture being the main factor to shape their behaviour. For example, one research participant reported crying and being distressed due to the decisions professionals made which she was not happy with despite the woman's attempt to express her wishes. But the professionals made a threat to stop her from expressing her feelings by telling her that social services could be contacted to take her baby away.

> I was crying in the corridor; the deputy head told me to stop otherwise she was going to tell social services to take my baby. I never saw her talk in that tone to anyone. I felt like what am I doing here. All I needed was accommodation, but I ended up getting medication.
>
> (p. 10)

> Africans we are despised, it takes a lot of confidence to be an African and the African mum. and especially living in such country and there is so much pressure.
>
> (Participant 4)

The women not talking openly about their experiences of racism maybe as a result of their upbringing as part of being an African woman which is next.

Being an African woman

Not all research participants talked openly about racism, and some internalised their experiences and associated this with harm. This tendency to internalise worsens a lack of understanding about the effects of cultural beliefs on perinatal mental ill-health. This may lead to integrate their experiences of racism into PNMHS.

> They brought a car, and they said you are going to mother and baby unit I said ooh my God, they're taking me to village where they will kill me. I was so scared, and I was just praying.
>
> (p. 3)

These women reported that since their childhood, they have been taught to remain strong and cope with any challenges which are part of being an African woman. This theme has been explained in detail in my findings. But the snapshot of it is that what shapes an African woman is her ability to deal with any obstacles and still stand strong as an African woman is regarded as the backbone of the family. For instance, one research participant narrated that:

> As an African woman I have to do everything for me, I felt like I had to be strong, hard-working and I cannot have a break like I have to be a superwoman.
>
> (p. 7)

Such cultural belief of being strong may have led these women not to talk openly about various issues including those around racism that they encounter during their journeys into PNMHS.

> Being an African woman is to be strong in managing a situation that you are in, to learn to cope to live around things at a young age you are able to cope with difficult situation and as you grow up you are able to continue coping.
>
> (Participant 10)

Immigration, colonialisation, and decolonisation

It is estimated that global migration involves over 286 million people of which nearly half are women, including those women of children-bearing age (The World Bank, 2011). There are various causes of global migration including political and socio-economic factors such as better employment opportunities, improved living standards, a family reunion in the country of destination, and studying (Castelli, 2018; Foner, 2009). Traditionally, men were a dominant group of migrants for work in a country of destination as women, who were dependents of men, were left behind to continue with family and household duties (Foner, 2009). But in the past four decades, women have equally been part of various migrant streams, which has led to a new migration movement and changes in paradigms in migration studies (Green, 2013; Holliday et al., 2019).

The increased number of human migrations to the west has led to hardening attitudes about migration (Migration Policy Institute, 2019), and altered relationships among sending, receiving, and transit countries as native populations of these countries express mixed views about migrations (Segal, 2019). There is evidence to show that migrants, particularly from ethnic minority background, do experience considerable resistance which includes racism from local natives (Weldon, 2006). However, non-western ethnicity and migration have been ignored or poorly conceptualised in contemporary scholarship, practice, policies including law, migration, health, and education (Erel et al., 2016; Scholten and Geddes, 2016).

Migration to the West can also be explained as the aftermath of colonisation (Bosma et al., 2012), the overall domination of European countries to the African continent based on power being in the hands of the western colonialists despite the resistance movements to counterbalance the invasion in many areas (Gueye, 2018). Western colonisation of Africa (in particular) in the 18th and 19th centuries divided societies into new boundaries and cultures different from the traditional societal way of living, the 'divide and rule' approach. This approach created political and social instability, as well as entrenched colonialisation of scholarship in this area. The dominance and supremacy of western scholars in matters pertaining to ethnicity, migration, culture, and race (Kaufmann and Haklai, 2008), elite institutions, publications, scholarships, and sponsorships have led to global knowledge-based experts' production and relations inequalities between western and non-western scholars (Kofman, 2020).

The colonial divide and rule approach is responsible for the formation of diverse cultural groups within countries in the Sub-Saharan African continent (Ocheni and Nwankwo, 2012). This explains the number of ethnic and cultural differences within nations within Sub-Saharan Africa. And the presence of African citizens with different ethnic backgrounds such as Asians, and indigenous Africans (Aixelà, 2013; Green, 2013). Nevertheless, Sub-Saharan Africa is used as a common identity for migrant women from a range of different ethnic and national backgrounds in the UK. What makes African migrant women a unique group from other ethnic groups in the United Kingdom is the fact that little is known about their lived experiences in the United Kingdom (Ochieng, 2012). As a group in the United Kingdom, they experience what might be seen as group challenges in accessing the available health services due to barriers such as structural and systemic racism, limited knowledge about access and availability of these services (Jankovic et al., 2020). On this matter, western scholars are urged to be self-reflective and move beyond the current western dominance in scholarship by being open and receptive to theories and models on race and ethnicity that emanate from different parts of the world (Suzuki, 2017). This includes decolonisation, promoting more studies on race and ethnicity away from the West, by accommodating indigenous knowledge research collaboratively carried out by researchers and participants from the same backgrounds (Keane et al., 2016) as knowledge generated in indigenous knowledge research should benefit and relate back to the lives of people in their respective communities by improving the quality of their lives. This growing impetus to develop diverse and inclusive knowledge away from the current western dominance is crucial in a bid to continue building inclusive multicultural societies in the West (Moreno and Chhatwal, 2020). The findings from my study resonate this as some research participants have reiterated the need for more research focusing the Sub-Saharan migrant women in UK as these women feel that little is known about their health needs. This group of migrant women suggested for researchers to come from the Sub-Saharan migrant group as they believe that new knowledge will be generated in a fair and trustworthy manner.

> I feel that a lot of research must be done within every ethnic background includes Sub-Saharan migrants as they will be able to get treatment that work for black people. Do you understand why there is a need for more research?
>
> (p. 2)

It is important to understand culturally diverse societies as it can be effective in tackling challenges faced by people with mental illness as it will reduce the cultural stigma that leads to the failure to talk openly about mental illness, it will help professionals in understanding symptoms of mental illness as described by individuals from an ethnic minority perspective, and it will help in exploring community resources available (Bhui et al., 2007).

Every society has its own cultural way of making sense of mental illness, describing the symptoms, and making use of coping strategies and support available (Fernando, 2011). Fernando specifically points out that ethnic minorities who are in the Western world have been affected by their home cultures. This may be a reason why they are less likely to accept and seek mental health treatment than other majority western societies. It is also important for health care professionals to be culturally sensitive and integrate some traditional ways such as that of consulting older family members and oracles in their respective communities when it comes to health decision matters (Omenka et al., 2020).

In culturally diverse western countries, mental health care systems need to be diverse and serve the needs of increasingly diverse populations. Therefore, understanding ethnic minority societies' perceptions about mental illness can be an effective step towards tackling their reluctance in accessing formal services (Brown et al., 1999). Most of research participants suggested for the increased number of people from black and ethnic backgrounds in higher positions as they feel that institutional racism starts from the top of hierarchy.

> I think a lot need to be done to support in the community and help people from ethnic minority background. We need to have more people from ethnic minority groups on a higher level to understand us. This is because those who are in the higher posts are not doing their job properly. They are the ones who are racist and do not care whether these women from Africa are suffering, they don't care at all.
>
> (p. 10)

Conclusions

To summarise, it appears that research participants found it difficult to talk about issues around racism and its discriminatory acts they faced when accessing British healthcare services. Either they are not informed, or they are used to be treated that way. Out of eleven research participants interviewed, three came forward to confirm having experienced both individual and structural racism. Seven of them needed prompts to describe what appeared to be discriminatory acts as the result of their colour of their skin. This led to assumption about their mental health and treatment and temporary separation from their babies as they felt treated differently. Temporary separation seemed to be another evidence of professionals' lack of urgency to understand and a treat Sub-Saharan African migrant women and the use of option of temporary separation and medication. The presence of formal means of detaining these women was used as protective factor by professionals to make such decisions which led to African migrant women's receipt treatment against their will. These narratives are similar to the tenets of CRT which also call for knowledge decolonisation in order to bring changes in perception about ethnic minorities and the concept of inequalities in health.

Note

1 If a woman has family, the baby will go to them. But if she does not have, children services arrange temporary fostering until a decision is made about the admission and whether the woman can be admitted to a mother and baby unit. This separation is temporary although some women reported being separated for up to three months which they found stressful.

References

Abbas, T., (2006). A question of reflexivity in a qualitative study of South Asians in education: Power, knowledge and shared ethnicity. *Ethnography and Education*, 1(3), pp.319–332.

Adebayo, C.T., Parcell, E.S., Mkandawire-Valhmu, L. and Olukotun, O., (2022). African American Women's maternal healthcare experiences: a Critical Race Theory perspective. *Health Communication*, 37(9), pp.1135–1146.

Ahmad, M., (2022). Care and migration: A reflexive account of a researcher with a migration background. *Qualitative Report, 27*(7), pp. 1341–1358. https://doi.org/10.46743/2160-3715/2022.5398

Aixelà, Y., (2013). Of colonists, migrants and national identity: The historic difficulties of the socio-political construction of Equatorial Guinea. *Nordic Journal of African Studies, 22*(1&2), pp.23–23.

Allan, H.T. and Arber, A., (2018). *Emotions and Reflexivity in Health and Social Care Field Research.* Gewerbestrasse: Palgrave Macmillan.

Bansal, N., Karlsen, S., Sashidharan, S.P., Cohen, R., Chew-Graham, C.A. and Malpass, A., (2022). U.nderstanding ethnic inequalities in mental healthcare in the UK: A meta-ethnography. *PLoS Medicine, 19*(12), p.e1004139.

Bergink, V., Laursen, T.M., Johansen, B.M.W., Kushner, S.A., Meltzer-Brody, S. and Munk-Olsen, T., (2015). Pre-clampsia and first-onset postpartum psychiatric episodes: A Danish population-based cohort study. *Psychological Medicine, 45*(16), 3481–3489.

Bhui, K., Warfa, N., Edonya, P., McKenzie, K. and Bhugra, D., (2007). Cultural competence in mental health care: A review of model evaluations. *BMC Health Services Research, 7*(1), pp.1–10.

Binder, P., Johnsdotter, S. and Essen, B., (2012). Conceptualising the prevention of adverse obstetric outcomes among immigrants using the three days framework in a high-income context. *Social Science & Medicine, 75*(11), 2028–2036 [Online]. Available from: https://doi.org/10.1016/j.socscimed.2012.08.010. Accessed on 9th May, 2021.

Bosma, U., Lucassen, J., Oostindie, G.J. and Oostindie, G., (eds), (2012). Introduction. Postcolonial migrations and identity politics: Towards a comparative perspective. In *Postcolonial Migrants and Identity Politics* (pp. 1–22). Publisher: Berghahn Books.

Brown, T.N., Sellers, S.L., Brown, K.T., Jackson, J.S., Aneshensel, C.S. and Phelan, J.C., (1999). Race, ethnicity, and culture in the sociology of mental health. In Aneshensel, C.S., Phelan, J.C. (eds), *Handbook of the Sociology of Mental Health* (pp. 167–182). Boston, MA: Springer.

Castelli, F., (2018). Drivers of migration: Why do people move? *Journal of Travel Medicine, 25*(1), p.tay040.

Christensen, T. and Lægreid, P., (eds), (2017). Introduction–theoretical approach and research questions. In *Transcending New Public Management* (pp. 13–28). London: Routledge.

Davies, C.A., (2008). *Reflexive Ethnography: A Guide to Researching Selves and Others.* London: Routledge.

Delgado, Richard and Stefancic, Jean, Critical Race Theory: An Annotated Bibliography (1993). Virginia Law Review, Vol. 79, 1993, U of Alabama Legal Studies Research Paper No. 2411618, Available at SSRN: https://ssrn.com/abstract=2411618

Delgado, R. and Stefancic, J., (2023). *Critical Race Theory: An Introduction* (Vol. 87). New York: NYU Press.

Department of Health, (2016). Department of Health annual report and accounts 2016 to 2017 – GOV.UK (www.gov.uk).

Erel, U., Murji, K. and Nahaboo, Z., (2016). Understanding the contemporary race–migration nexus. *Ethnic and Racial Studies, 39*(8), pp.1339–1360.

Fernando, S., (2011). A 'global' mental health program or markets for Big Pharma. *Nature, 475,* pp.27–30.

Foner, N. ed., (2009). *Across Generations: Immigrant Families in America.* New York: NYU Press.

Giorgi, A., (2012). The descriptive phenomenological psychological method. *Journal of Phenomenological Psychology, 43*(1), 3–12.

Green, N.L., (2013). Donna R. Gabaccia and Mary Jo Maynes (eds), Changing paradigms in migration studies: From men to women to gender. *Gender History Across Epistemologies*, pp.262–278.

Gueye, M., (2018). Colonialism in Africa: A revisionist perspective. *Africology: The Journal of Pan African Studies, 12*(1), pp.111–122.

Helberg-Proctor, A., Meershoek, A., Krumeich, A. and Horstman, K., (2017). 'Foreigners','ethnic minorities', and 'non-Western allochtoons': An analysis of the development of 'ethnicity' in health policy in the Netherlands from 1970 to 2015. *BMC Public Health, 17*(1), pp.1–13.

Holliday, J., Hennebry, J. and Gammage, S., (2019). Achieving the sustainable development goals: Surfacing the role for a gender analytic of migration. *Journal of Ethnic and Migration Studies, 45*(14), pp.2551–2565.

Huddle, T.S., (2022). Against the turn to critical race theory and "anti-racism" in academic medicine. In *HEC Forum* (pp. 1–20). Dordrecht: Springer.

Jankovic, J., Parsons, J., Jovanović, N. et al. (2020). Differences in access and utilisation of mental health services in the perinatal period for women from ethnic minorities—a population-based study. *BMC Medicine 18*, pp. 245. https://doi.org/10.1186/s12916-020-01711-w

Joseph, F.I., Earland, J. and Ahmed, M.A., (2021). Experience of conducting sensitive qualitative research as a cultural outsider: Formulation of a guide for reflexivity. *International Journal of Qualitative Methods, 20*, p.16094069211058616.

Karisen, S. and Nazroo, J.Y., (2002). Relation between racial discrimination, social class, and health among ethnic minority groups. *American Journal of Public Health, 92*(4), pp.624–631. [Online]. Available from: https://ajph.aphapublications.org/doi/10.2105/AJPH.92.4.624. Accessed on 29th April, 2002.

Kaufmann, E. and Haklai, O., (2008). Dominant ethnicity: From minority to majority. *Nations and Nationalism, 14*(4), pp.743–767.

Keane, M., Constance, K., and Muza, B. 2016. It matters who you are: indigenous knowledge research and researchers. *Education as Change, 20*(2), pp.163–183. https://doi.org/10.17159/1947-9417/2016/913

Kerstetter, K., (2012). Insider, outsider, or somewhere between: The impact of researchers' identities on the community-based research process. *Journal of Rural Social Sciences, 27*(2), p.7.

Kofman, E., (2020). Unequal internationalisation and the emergence of a new epistemic community: Gender and migration. *Comparative Migration Studies, 8*(1), pp.1–6.

Latif, Z., (2014). A Race Equality Foundation Briefing Paper: Better Health Briefing 31: The maternal mental health of migrant women. [Online]. Available from: https://www.better-health.org.uk. Accessed on 23rd March, 2019.

Ling, L., Eraso, Y. and Mascio, V.D., (2023). First-generation Nigerian mothers living in the UK and their experience of postnatal depression: An interpretative phenomenological analysis. *Ethnicity & Health, 28*(5), pp.738–756.

Migration Policy Institute, (2019). Migration Policy Institute | migrationpolicy.org

Moreno, F.A. and Chhatwal, J., (2020). Diversity and inclusion in psychiatry: The pursuit of health equity. *Focus, 18*(1), pp.2–7.

National Collaborating Centre for Mental Health, National Institute for Health, Clinical Excellence, British Psychological Society and Royal College of Psychiatrists, (2011). *Common Mental Health Disorders: Identification and Pathways to Care*. London: NICE.

National Institute for Health and Care Excellence (2014) Antenatal and postnatal mental health: clinical management and service guidance. Clinical guideline Published: 17 December 2014 Last updated: 11 February 2020. Accesssed 17th August 2023. https://www.nice.org.uk/guidance/cg192

NHS Digital, (2021). Mental Health Act Statistics, Annual Figures, 2021-22 – NDRS (digital.nhs.uk).

NHS UK, (2019). NHS Long Term Plan » The NHS Long Term Plan.

NICE, (2016). Guidance, NICE Advice and Quality Standards. Available from https://www.nice.org.uk/guidance/published?from=2016-11-01&to=2016-11-30. Accessed on 23rd December, 2022.

Ocheni, S. and Nwankwo, B.C., (2012). Analysis of colonialism and its impact in Africa. *Journal of Cross Cultural Communication, 8*(3), pp.46–54. [Online]. Available from: https://www.doi:10.3968/j.ccc.1923670020120803.1189. Accessed on 02nd March, 2022.

Ochieng BMN, (2012). Black African migrants: The barriers with accessing and utilizing health promotion services in the UK. *European Journal of Public Health, 23*(2), pp.265–269.

Omenka, O.I., Watson, D.P. and Hendrie, H.C., (2020). Understanding the healthcare experiences and needs of African immigrants in the United States: A scoping review. *BMC Public Health, 20,* pp.1–13.

Palaniappan, K. and Kum, I.Y.S., (2019). Underlying causes behind research study participants' careless and biased responses in the field of sciences. *Current Psychology, 38*(6), pp.1737–1747.

Pangas, J., Ogunsiji, O., Elmir, R., Raman, S., Liamputtong, P., Burns, E., Dahlen, H.G. and Schmied, V., (2019). Refugee women's experiences negotiating motherhood and maternity care in a new country: A meta-ethnographic review. *International Journal of Nursing Studies, 90,* pp.31–45.

Pilav, S., Easter, A., Silverio, S.A., De Backer, K., Sundaresh, S., Roberts, S. and Howard, L.M., (2022). Experiences of perinatal mental health care among minority ethnic women during the COVID-19 pandemic in London: A qualitative study. *International Journal of Environmental Research and Public Health, 19*(4), p.1975.

Pitard, J., (2017), September. A journey to the centre of self: Positioning the researcher in autoethnography. In *Forum Qualitative Sozialforschung/Forum: Qualitative Social Research* (Vol. 18, No. 3, pp. 1–20).

Reiners, G.M., (2012). Understanding the differences between Husserl's (descriptive) and Heidegger's (interpretive) phenomenological research. *Journal of Nursing & Care, 1*(5), pp.1–3.

Scholten, P. and Geddes, A., (2016). The politics of migration and immigration in Europe. In *The Politics of Migration and Immigration in Europe*. London: Sage.

Segal, U.A., (2019). Globalization, migration, and ethnicity. *Public Health, 172,* pp.135–142.

Smith, M.S., Lawrence, V., Sadler, E. and Easter, A., (2019). Barriers to accessing mental health services for women with perinatal mental illness: Systematic review and meta-synthesis of qualitative studies in the UK. *BMJ Open, 9*(1), p.e024803.

Suzuki, K., (2017). A critical assessment of comparative sociology of race and ethnicity. *Sociology of Race and Ethnicity*, 3(3), pp.287–300.

The Royal College of Psychiatrists, (2018). Mental health in pregnancy. November 2018. Available from: https://www.rcpsych.ac.uk/.../college-reports/2018-college-reports. Accessed 17th August 2023.

Weldon, S.A., (2006). The institutional context of tolerance for ethnic minorities: A comparative, multilevel analysis of Western Europe. *American Journal of Political Science*, 50(2), pp.331–349.

World Bank, (2011). *World Development Report 2011: Conflict, Security, and Development*. The World Bank.

World Health Organisation, (2017). Adolescents and mental health. [Online]. Available from: https:// www.who.int/maternal-child-adolescent/topics/adolescence/mental-health/en. Accessed on 6th February, 2019.

World Health Organization, (2018). Improving the health care of pregnant refugee and migrant women and newborn children. [Online]. Available from: https://iris.who.int/handle/10665/342289. Accessed on 4th May, 2021.

5 An ethnography of Islamophobia

David Ring

Introduction

I undertook research into the experiences of Muslims studying nursing in London using ethnography. My PhD was concerned with the place of Muslims in a wider non-Muslim society. I am a white, English, Christian, heterosexual man which required me to explicitly reflect on my position(ality), my research methodology, methods and analytic devices to support the authenticity and truthfulness of my data and its analysis. In short, to justify, how I, a powerful outsider from such distance, may truthfully and ethically be able to research the experiences of a minoritised group of people.

Research should be undertaken with a considered methodology and data does not by "common sense" give meaning, as every stage is underpinned by reflexive use of theory (Braun and Clarke, 2022). This chapter focuses on the reflexivity used throughout. I start with a discussion of the nature of the society in which the participants exist, that is, the overarching contextual structure. I discuss my epistemological position (how one shows that one knows reality) and how positionality, reflection and reflexivity were all integral to my research. I then examine the individual participants' experiences and micro-sociological interactions reflexively, that is by reflecting on how reflexivity shaped the findings. I do not intend to present the findings as such, but focus entirely on the reflexivity which was essential to analysing the data. I focus on intersectionality to discuss six experiences of fieldwork; faith, diet, race/ethnicity, social class, sex/gender and age. Finally, symbolic interactionism (Goffman, 1959, 1963; Rock, 2001) informed by intersectionality theory (Crenshaw, 1989; Collins and Bilge, 2020) and critical race theory (Gholami, 2021), as analytical devices for a thematic analysis of the data and presentation of findings are reflected on. I discuss how I used my insider/outsider statuses and self-disclosure to varying degrees as tools to aid the practice of reflexivity in relation to the findings.

The research project and me

I registered as a nurse in January 1992, and have a background in palliative care; I am a lecturer in nursing at Middlesex University in north London. I have led many and varied modules during this time and I began to notice

DOI: 10.4324/9781003269915-5

that year three Muslim nursing students regularly reflected upon experiences of racism and Islamophobia that they faced while undergraduates when given the opportunity. I decided to investigate their experiences.

After considering many research approaches I decided to undertake an ethnographic project using participant observation of self-identified Muslim undergraduate nursing students. I spent several months accompanying students from when they left their homes in the mornings, to when they returned home, however late, while they were in the academic parts of their studies. This type of ethnography involved participating in the direct experiences of participants as they travelled, attended lessons, met in study groups, attended prayers, fasted and socialised. My field notes (over 70,000 words) were generated by observing events, asking questions and feeding back to the participants and their peers. The collection and analysis of data are being used to submit for a PhD degree in nursing.

While in the role of researcher as a nurse, I had to pay attention to, and abide by the NMC Code (Nursing and Midwifery Council, 2018). I was also a lecturer at the institution at which the participants and their peers were undergraduates and I needed to be aware of the power imbalance and of a possible Hawthorne effect. The former was an ongoing issue but the latter was quickly overcome. The Hawthorne effect, also known as the observer effect, is the idea that when knowingly observed, those being watched might change their behaviour. This is based upon a non-participant study in the 1920s in a glass factory in the USA. Paradis and Sutkin (2016) argue that there is no evidence it truly occurs substantially, that it is just a "good story." If participants and the observed do change their behaviour then it is very minor and only for a short time. In my field work the students became very open and candid very quickly, openly discussing staff, colleagues, peers and their personal lives candidly and at length, to such an extent that I felt I needed to retain confidences.

Ethnography is the methodological approach which facilitates a researcher to tell a person or group of people's stories through their own eyes rather than the researcher's (Vindrola-Padros, 2021). Its methods involve the researcher immersing themselves into the practices and lives of a group of people existing within a society. It aims to explicitly examine their experiences and their understandings of the relationships between their culture and behaviours (Gray, 2014 adapting Tesch, 1994) within the context of their environment. The method I used is participant observation where the researcher immerses themselves in the everyday lives of the participants; this involves, watching, listening, noting, reflecting feeding back and conducting ethnographic interviews in the field (Spradley, 1975) and the "waiting field" (Folkes, 2022). The field (Coffey, 1999) being the classic idea of where research takes place, when research is consciously being undertaken, but the "waiting field" as identified by Folkes (2022) involves the non-specific, case dependent margins. In my project the field was me accompanying the participants in their daily activities while the waiting field included the times that participants and non-participants came and found me in my office, or when teaching, when having my lunch, and supplied me with data they wanted included. At such times the location was different, my mindset was different, and I began to carry a blank hardback note book separately to record such meetings. I was aware of a dynamic insider or outsider dichotomy (Ademolu, 2023) and the need to be explicitly reflexive on positionality throughout (Merton, cited by Coser, 1975; Alejandro, 2023).

In order to produce an ethnography, to tell another's story, one has to learn the practice of walking in another person's shoes (Riessman, 2007) in as disinterested a fashion as possible to deliver some analysable representations of "authentic" truths; of valid knowledge (Ademolu, 2023). The researcher is telling a story (Geertz, 1973) from a viewpoint, a position and the acknowledgement of this and its effect on how the data are produced and processed are key methodological issues of epistemology that require identifying and analysing. The context within which the social activities take place needs to be described and evaluated too.

The researcher needs to strike a balance between reflexivity as a tool to interrogate and validate the work produced without over-centring themselves. Said (1978) indicates that one cannot begin to know another until one knows oneself and Pillow (2003) tempers this by warning that in the attempt to be a non-exploitative and credible researcher one may slide into self-indulgence, or worse, narcissism. This chapter looks at the theoretical underpinnings of how I, as far an outsider as almost could be, was able to show authenticity in the research process. This will be done by showing position and how biases are inevitable (Haraway, 1991) as social realities and how theories of epistemological, positionality, reflection, reflexivity can be used to overcome the challenges of intersectional distance and difference; in short, how a privileged white man can attempt to present the story of minoritised Black and Brown Muslims.

The context for the study

Although widespread research shows Muslims, particularly Hijab wearing women (Bhatti, 2021) as being the recipients of a high level of discrimination (and at all gradations of discrimination), there is little on campus research experience of Islamophobia. Mir (2014) has researched the experience of Muslim women on US campuses and told compelling stories of undergraduates enduring discrimination while negotiating their identities. But this work is difficult to apply to the UK. In the US Muslims make up a smaller part of the student body and make up smaller proportions across universities (4% for Mir, 2014). Figures for religion are not collated as accurately as for ethnicity in the UK but using what was available (Malik and Wykes, 2018) it appears that numbers are higher across the HE sector. The university in which my project took place is 71% Black and Brown overall and in the nursing department 91% BAME (2020, when this term was used) and approximately 20%

Muslim. The effect here is that the Muslim nursing students are not isolated and outnumbered as their US counterparts and thus pressured to integrate and be cross-examined as spokespeople for Muslims.

Society in the UK is one of white male Christian supremacy. Morrison (2019) states that proving racism (and other oppressions) is a distraction, a "one more thing," circle that can never end. That those who benefit from the structural inequality of a society have the social capital to endlessly ask for evidence by reshaping questions, by asking new questions, by asking for newer material because were it to be accepted then these highly successful but "mediocre white men" (Eddo-Lodge, 2017) might have to accept that their success was not based on talent alone; that there is a cultural need for a belief in a functioning meritocracy. The explanation of the first statement here must be seen within that context; the committed racist will never acknowledge the racism.

Nonetheless, the setting for my research is such a society and justification for this viewpoint is required. This can be done first by exploring its meaning. Fleming (2019) makes the point polemically, that part of the culture which maintains white supremacy is that it works to ensure that we are "stupid about race." Lentin (2020) calls this a lack of "racial literacy," an inability to think critically about race. She gives the example of people overlooking power structures, and in doing so, confusing any kind of prejudice or bigotry with racism. Collins (2015) explains that the history told is that of white, propertied men, that we (I am one) are seen as the "normal, the universal" type (Garner, 2007; Morrison, 2017; Sue, 2015; Bonilla-Silva, 2021). This white universalism is unspoken, unanalysed and unchallenged (DiAngelo, 2019). Bell's (1992) second rule of racial standing is that Black people are unable to speak of racism because they are biased as a result of being involved negatively, and that only white researchers and commentators may speak and judge objectively. Najib (2022) adapts this to Islamophobia stating how in French academia being a Muslim is seen as a disadvantage in studying Muslims because only a (white) outsider can offer objectivity. White supremacy here means that there is an often unspoken (a cultural hegemonic) facet of the UK that the default setting is white and male and that this is structural (Hall, 2021). Having representation does not change this for a Black or Brown person may come to unreflexively practise the supremacy of white maleness, by internalising the system and upholding it. They may do this unaware that they are upholding white male supremacy.

White male supremacy oppresses women. Rosalind Franklin, Caroline Herschel, Lise Meitner, Hertha Ayrton, Marietta Blau and Henderina Scott illustrate examples of the invisibility of women. They were all high achieving women who made major contributions in the natural sciences that resulted in awards and fame for their male collaborators but little for them. Rossiter (1993) has described this as the "Matilda effect," a fate shared by one of UK's nursing founders, Mary Seacole, but for her Blackness rather than her femaleness.

White male hegemony in British society is evident in its leaders and their religious affiliation. Firstly, the British monarch is "Defender of the Faith"; that faith, of course, is the Anglican Church, whose senior clergy are awarded seats in the House of Lords, which has significant symbolic and political power. Secondly, senior British judges (high court and above), the largest group, describe themselves as Church of England (35%), the next largest having "no religion" (34%), with 15% identifying as Jewish and 4.3% as Muslim at (high court level only) and none recorded as Roman Catholic. Of these senior judges, only four percent are Black or Brown (Ministry of Justice, 2022). When Munby (2013) declares the judiciary to be secular, his meaning is clearly an undeclared Protestant idea of secularity. The UK is unthinkingly hegemonically Anglican, just as it is white and male.

The white male supremacy of the UK does not mean that society is an overtly, individually racist and Islamophobic one (although Muslims may and do receive individualised actions of open racism and Islamophobia) but that it is institutionally so (MacPherson, 1999). The research participants exist in a macro environment that is detrimental to them in that it is Islamophobic (Runnymede, 1997, 2016; All Party Parliamentary Group on British Muslims [APPG], 2018) and that this is intersectionally enhanced by Muslims being racialised in a minoritising way (Moosavi, 2014; APPG, 2018).

Reflexivity and positionality explored

In order to practise reflexivity, it is necessary to identify and define positionality. Alejandro (2023) defines this as asking *who* is speaking, from *where* and finally *how* (his italics) they are doing so. Collins (2015) and Collins and Bilge (2016, 2020) offer a list of sociological identities that interact to produce intersectional discrimination and "as a way of understanding and analysing complexity in the world" (2016, p. 25). These lend themselves to the researcher asking *who I am*, from *where I am* speaking and recognising that a singular identity involves multiple viewpoints. Together with Crenshaw (1995) the identities are labelled as ethnicity/race, gender, social class/status, citizenship, age, (dis)ability, sexuality and religion. Collins and Bilge (2020) make clear that inequality, social context and power relationships are intrinsic parts of these features; they are not a simple checklist but an interacting set of narratives tied to identity.

Reyes (2020) indicates how the researchers' status, and locations on this list effect everything about ethnography from data collection, to its writing up, analysing and authority. She highlights how power and social capital are inseparable from this list in that membership of each identity group includes such features. The list of categories is dynamic; they change in meaning and number (religion and disability being recent additions) and the researcher is not fixed within them; they move between over time and in certain situations. Reyes (2020) shows how while her ethnicity has remained static its position in a hierarchy changes and that her social class position has changed considerably as she has gained in status and wealth via career success. Folkes (2022), in agreement, notes that engagement should not be checking of items on a "shopping list," as if completed, but that they require ongoing engagement. She adds that some are visible, such as race and gender, while others are invisible. Some fall between and some move between. For example, our characters, personalities, our life experiences, our childhoods, our social origins are largely invisible (and may evolve) or require much skill and attention to perceive them. Our race and gender are visible. Our social class may be either, as social class is, via our use of symbols, possible to perceive (Goffman, 1959). Bourdieu (1977) states that our taste is a product of our class and we subconsciously use it to communicate to the world who we are; for example, the coat we choose may be for warmth but it always a symbol of taste which is a class indicator. Religion can be both visible (a hijab and abaya signs of Muslimness or Jesus on a cross is Catholic) and invisible (class). And of course, religion can have meaning as a manifestation of social class.

In shopping list fashion (Folkes, 2022), I can add categories to Collins and Bilge's (2020) list as I identify as a white, Christian, middle-class, heterosexual, vegetarian man in my fifties with comparative wealth and social capital. I come from a family where no one has/had been to university and was raised in a subculture where only the occasional religious leader had received a higher education. I was raised in a part of Essex that was near universally white and made up of east London, working class "white flighters." Anderson (2022) explains "white flight" as a long-term dynamic process of white people vacating neighbourhood when the perceive an "invasion and succession" occurring as an imprecise number of Black people move to the area, and they wish to avoid living alongside them Kaufmann and Harris (2015) document this process occurring widely in the UK but argue that it is caused less by race or racism but more by an attraction to where the movers have migrated to; towards economic betterment. Either way, the outcome was white people leaving east London in large numbers in the 1960s and 1970s and moving to south east Essex.

Pillow (2003) states that reflexivity is more precisely self-reflexivity and differs from reflection in that there must an 'other' and that there must be a self-conscious scrutiny of the self and awareness of the process. Haraway (1991) suggests that an explicit and open questioning of self and one's relationships with the research project is a process in itself that leads towards a form of objectivity by intelligent candour. I am kind, approachable, funny, intellectual, intermittently situationally socially awkward, mildly obsessive, and perpetually badly dressed. The ongoing reflexivity has also changed my perceptions of *who* I am and *how* I interact. I wish to avoid the narcissistic, self-indulgent look at myself, but only the reader can judge if I have overstepped into the territory humorously indicated by Marcus (1999, citing Stacey, 1990), "as the Fijian said to the new ethnographer, 'that's enough talking about you; let's talk about me.'" This is not about me but I have to be present, to interrogate that presence, in order for the reader to judge for authenticity and truth of my work.

Reyes (2020) and Folkes (2022) both used self-disclosure of their invisible positions to engender trust and revelations from their participants. The former in terms of her childhood and origins; she may appear as a middle-class academic researcher, possessed of social capital but her childhood was poor, low status, fractured and shared many of the disadvantaged characteristics of her participants as well as their ethnicity and religion. The latter, Folkes (2022) revealed that she shared a lower working-class background from a similar (and very pertinently for her research) geographical origin. These are invisible positions, dynamic features that have altered as the researchers have moved up the social ladder. It is reflexivity that leads to self-disclosure and reflexivity that leads one to know oneself and identify what is relevant.

It is, therefore necessary for me to be reflexive on my journey to validate my data, its collection and analysis. I am an invisibly different person now from the one who began this project. Before nursing I studied sociology and minored in philosophy, at an old and traditional university and choose the options available that brought most overlap, particularly the philosophy of sociology and the sociology of religion. I had a very religious non-conformist Protestant upbringing and questions of faith have remained central to how I think and make decisions. The study of Descartes and Goffman as an undergraduate particularly left habits of thought in me about Cartesian ideas of duality, of mind-body separation, and of epistemology; these have returned during my PhD and I draw on them as I see them as relevant. Descartes's ideas that to doubt, to debate oneself, is the proof of consciousness and free existence are particularly pertinent. Constant self-doubt and self-questioning are habits that have increased as I have progressed through my PhD. The importance of the categories that make up who I am and their shifts in importance tally well with the modern positionality literature here, notable Folkes (2022), Alejandro (2023), Pillow, (2003) and Reyes (2020).

I will work through the key categories in the findings from my study that required reflexivity and shall begin with the ones that helped me connect to the participants. In order of being addressed these are: faith and religion, diet, social class, race, sex/gender and age. They are mediated by self-disclosure which has an effect of transcending positional categories (Folkes, 2022). Self-disclosure allows problematisation of one's positionality which enables the subconscious to be made explicit and for the question, "by what right?" to be debated (Alejandro, 2021). There is a benefit on being an outsider and knowing less because the insider/outsider dichotomy is problematic in itself. As Ademolu (2023) notes as a Nigerian researching Nigerian groups, his similarity at times bred suspicion and possibly detrimental over-familiarity. In contrast at certain times, "critical junctions" (Alejandro, 2021) an outsider may be seen as distanced and this perceived as a disinterest that enables curiosity to triumph over perceived judgement.

Six fieldwork experiences giving rise to reflexivity; faith, diet as culture, race, class, sex/gender and age

A prominent feature of the fieldwork was faith. Faith, not religion, not its individual practice but a belief in the metaphysical, in religious texts as life manuals and the *a priori* ideas of deontological ethics, was a substantial experience of everyday life for the participants and importantly, a substantial and unexpected connection for me with the Muslim students. All participants stated a doubt-free belief in God, regardless of how orthopraxically they behaved or how centrally they placed the practice of Islam in their lives. This was a bonding category and a commonality that was explicitly told to me. For example, with all of the participants we discussed faith, religion and how they impact upon life decisions; for those of any faith negotiating an ostensibly and self-declared secular society is an ongoing challenge. This experience connected me to the participants as they used the same but differently named God and a different prophet to guide them from the one I use. The approach to life decisions we shared in these discussions was (I am wondering) about how to lead my life and refer back to faith.

Wary of the self-indulgence potential here, this process clarified for me how strong my faith is, how its unrealised centrality is in my life and my need to attend to it. I have no particular interest in Islam itself, my work is not theology but one underpinning concern of mine is that people should be free and that one tenet of this is the freedom to practise (or not practise) their chosen religion (Foreign, Commonwealth and Development Office, 2022). I engaged in discussions with the participants about faith and religion; this was instigated by them and was caused by their willingness to share their faith and to hear about mine. The process involved me learning about Islam and my own positions and led me to realise that although I began by seeing my stance on Islam as neutral this was far from the truth; I had unconsciously absorbed much from the media and held stereotypical and frequently factually wrong ideas. One example being that I believed that any Muslim women who wore hijab and certainly any who wore jilbab/abaya would be a pious and enthusiastic practitioner of their faith. This proved to be an unfounded belief, an assumed preconception, because many women dressed that way for cultural reasons, ease of decision-making and (in Yasmiin's case) as a reaction to Islamophobia. As one said, "you hate Muslims, well then, I am going to be very fucking Muslim" (Yasmiin, participant).

Marcus (1986) states that reality is a social construction and that the reality engendered by research is one that is constructed in a manner specific to its methodology and methods. Research 'reality' means that there is a narrative apparatus used to represent the researcher's experience of the participants' reality and that the researcher should reflect on the techniques and how they relate to the production of the data. Historically in ethnography Marcus (1986) has posited that researchers have failed to so this. For example, Geertz (1973) produced a seminal piece of work on Muslims but rarely and without any evident theoretical structure to his thinking (it was there, but largely implicit) does he show any reflexivity on who he was; he assumed himself to be neutral (Varisco, 2005). The relevance here is that in discussing religion I was engaged in self-disclosure, a two-way learning process and the building of and deepening of ongoing relationships. Coffey (1999) indicates how the relationships between researcher and participants are relational and interactive, not abstract and that they in themselves effect the data produced and the techniques involved. Differences and the reflexivity of the researcher should be uncomfortable (Pillow, 2003) and this discomfort needs to be more than acknowledged. Kleinmann and Copp (1993) are clear that, for example, we must acknowledge whether we like or dislike our participants and that these feelings are part of the data. What this means here is that in discussing religion I do/did have thoughts on Islam and its validity, I am not neutral and to downplay this is to fall into the non-reflexive trap of the imperialist, Orientalist anthropologist of whom Said (1978) and Marcus (1986) speak.

Fundamentally, the nature of faith was an insider aspect of the project and many participants openly said this to me. They described that seeing in my online biography that I practise a faith was a deciding factor in allowing me to share their days. Several of the women renamed me "Da'ud" (Arabic for David), and the younger women started to call me "uncle Da'ud." Several said to me that, "once you find out just how great Islam is, you'll revert/ convert before you know it!" My positionality is an interactive, dynamic one that has an underpinning element but one that also changes and required on-going reflexivity. This might be a long way around saying the uncomfortable truth that I am/was Islamophobic myself. I have a set idea of my Christianity and an exegesis that I see as correct (for me). I had preconceived ideas about what Islam is and whether or not I approve; a subconscious position as I un-knowingly set myself up as a central narrator of the reality I was portraying. Van Loon (2001) makes the point that ethnography can have no central nar-rator, no "authority" because this is an attempt to make the temporary and contingent into the fixed and permanent; I came to realise that I was always interpreting and that my goal is to imperfectly attempt to represent a partial truth only.

One main participant was a Niqab-wearing woman, Kemi; the only part of her I could see was her eyes. I told myself that this was entirely her choice and that I had no feelings on the matter. In truth I am judgemental and do think ways of behaving have hierarchies. Spending time with Kemi was instructive in me reflecting upon *who* I am, *how* I think about representations of faith and gender (which follows later) as well as how I express these thoughts and how the language and structures I have available have effects (Alejandro, 2021). I was straining for a non-judgemental neutrality and fooling myself because I knew, even then, that even the language of such ideas was a reality-creating tool. Kemi's wearing of the Niqab was a recent (one year) change and something that she was not committed to long term; she saw it as part of her spiritual journey, a tool for now but not forever. The religious discussions between us involved shifting the dynamics and my position; to be reflexive one has to be very open to questions of psychodynamics (Hunt, 1989) and to one's biases.

The second important experience of fieldwork was a largely invisible one that Reyes (2020) calls a commonality to let the researcher into something shared that humanises and suggest to the participants that the researcher is in this particular way similar to them. This aspect of fieldwork was the cultural experience of diet. Interacting within my social class milieu I kept and keep quiet about my vegetarianism because it was unusual and I perceived it to be deemed unmanly and embarrassingly middle class in a proudly and pervasively working-class environment. When I became a vegetarian, it was perceived by many I knew with homophobia; not eating meat was verbalised (ostensibly humorously) as an obvious sign of homosexuality and that this was an undesirable quality. Within the field and between fields (Folkes, 2022) my vegetarianism was seen as a positive sign. For example, I remember having a chicken shop lunch with a group of women and awkwardly asking the man behind the counter about whether the oil used for the meat and fish was separate from that for the chips. It was not and so I had to sit foodless while everyone else ate. This, however, was remarked upon and discussed by the participants and their friends. They verbalised understanding and stated that they admired me for it; they said that it was similar to the halal food quest; a public naming of oneself as an outsider, a marginal. There are differences because I am a white man with all the power that that entails; in all the intersections I am much higher up the hierarchy while they are actively discriminated against. Nonetheless, my diet was perceived by the participants as an insider (Coffey, 1999) trait, a way to understand the insider position and culture, and an advantage in the research process; different but similar, a second small commonality in a sea of unequal difference.

The third experience which was profoundly shaped by my reflexivity in the data analysis is race; I am a white English man and all of the participants were Black or Brown people. There is no hierarchy of racisms or categories but dark-skinned Black people usually find themselves at the top of the discrimination ladder. Gillborn (2015) argues that there is no universal, unchanging ranking of discriminations but that overall being Black is the most disadvantageous in the UK. McCall (2005) explains how generally being a Black woman increases the level of discrimination and disadvantage faced but that this is not universal; there are circumstances under which being a Black man puts one higher up the hierarchy than being a Black woman, for example, the likelihood of being stopped and searched by the police in London. Race, or ethnicity are inseparable from the other categories overall but there are issues specific to perceived race that can be examined here. Certainly, my whiteness is a clear and obvious difference that distances me and categorically stops me from being able walk in the participants' shoes (Riessman, 2007). I am unequivocally unable to represent the perception of the participants' realities on race grounds alone, it is impossible. This is a state-ment of reality that threads through my work as a simple truth that has his-torically been missing from anthropologists' and ethnographers' works; but modern ethnographers note, I am telling only a partial truth (Clifford, 1986). Jackson (1989) notes that an ethnographer is attempting to write history as it is being lived, an impossible task. This does not invalidate the research, it is a caveat; the open, theory-based reflexivity enables the reader to see that the process has been robust and that the data and conclusions drawn are deeply considered and not claiming to be something that they are not.

Defining race is a complex and "travelling" (Goldberg, 2023) debate, it is a social construction that has evolved to manage human difference and maintain white supremacy (Lentin, 2020). Groups of people are racialised and then minoritised based on their racial ascription (Rollock, 2022). This is not the chapter to engage on the shifting meaning of races, Blackness, Brown-ness and what constitutes whiteness (Clarke and Garner, 2010), but a look at reflexivity and how a white researcher may attempt to represent a version, a partial truth of the experience of a minoritised group. This is a visible element of reflexivity in that the participants were South Asian and Black African in origin. They were mostly visibly Muslim too so this is practicably inseparable in terms of intersectionality. The insider/outsider concept can be defined as whether or not the researcher is a member of the group being studied (Braun and Clarke, 2021) and in this case, I am an outsider; I am neither Muslim nor a person of colour. There are complexities and nuances to what is an insider because of the multi-categorical nature of people. Reyes (2020), for example, visibly shares ethnic origin with her participants but differs in almost every other way, whereas Folkes (2022) invisibly shares social class and geographi-cal origins with her participants but again is otherwise different and needed to self-reveal that she shared such origins. This nuanced insider/outsider de-tail shows how there are gradations of otherness. One of my participants told me of the "type" of person his community labelled "Dagenham Dave," an archetypal Essex man whose characteristics I shared almost completely in origin but because I presented as a London-dwelling, middle class academic he was shocked to discover my origins.

Braun and Clarke (2021) argue that outsider status is an inadequate modi-fier. I am white and Protestant and these are both heavily laden with cul-tural potency, meaning and power. I am not just an outsider but an outsider with power looking in on a marginalised powerless group. This does not undermine the project but it needs reflexivity based on theory to show that I, the researcher, am aware of this and how the distance effects the research process. In short, I am producing a powerful white male, Christian filtering of the participants' voices. This filtering is not wholly negative because the complexities in this concept have advantages too; the outsider asks questions that the insiders may not see; "is that racist? Is that Islamophobic?" I fre-quently asked and the participants were so used to such events that they had ceased to consciously register them even though their behaviour was affected. For example, the hijab and jilbab-wearing women never looked up when seated on the underground and thought that people glaring at them with obvious hostility was "just" an everyday experience. I, on the other hand, believed that what I observed was racism. Further participants acknowledged my power and welcomed my interest; stating that if a white man like me elucidates the Islamophobia they face then people will acknowledge it as real in a way they do not when the marginalised complain. There are many caveats, conditions, complexities and ethical issues here so I am not simply "giving voice" (Braun and Clarke, 2021) to a group but a version of a voice is being promoted.

The final facet of the insider/outsider concept that needs exposition here is that the idea of an insider group is reductionist; it implies a degree of homogeneity that does not exist in reality. Hammersley and Atkinson (2007), writing about research on working class boys, argue that such participants do not represent a whole group and it is a mistake to see it as such and that robust ethnography makes no such claim. Further, the developing relationship between the participants and researcher has an impact. Ademolu (2023) writes of being part of the Nigerian diaspora that he researched how "birds of a feather don't always flock together." That simply because there are shared characteristics does not mean commonality and understanding. The diaspora is diverse and even when there are similarities he cites Simmel and Kurt (Ademolu, 2023, citing Simmel and Kurt, 1950) who query the whole concept, "one who is close by may be far and ...one who is remote is near." Further they state that an outsider may reverse acculturate and gain insight in a conscious way, rather than simply losing themselves and "going native." The latter is illustrated by Rock (2001) citing the examples of ethnographers of the police who have subsequently themselves enlisted and sociologists of religion who have converted during research on evangelical crusades. I presented some findings at an Islamic studies conference and realised during the questioning that many in the audience thought that I was a revert/convert, an insider of sorts. During the post-presentation discussion, it became clear Muslim researchers who researched Muslims felt that my outsider status acted as "fresh eyes" as long as I was vigilant of my status and privilege.

The fourth experience is social class, or socio-economic status. Social class here being understood as an individual's relationship to the means of production (owning, managing or labouring) combined with one's social standing; the classic Marx, adapted by Weber's interpretation (Giddens and Sutton, 2021). In practice this may be based on the UK government's "occupation stratification" (formerly the Registrar General's) model using specific occupations. In these systems background is irrelevant, current position is the over-riding feature and I am social class one as a lecturer or two as a registered nurse (Office for National Statistics, 2022). As with the other categories this is a nuanced one, dissected by the other traits and is fluid. However, the participants were all social class four and five, from working class families.

One non-participant who was regularly involved from the margins was a Somali woman who explained that her background was "bourgeois" as she was a senior politician's daughter, raised in wealth and with education until his assassination and her flight to Europe.

The fifth experience is gender/sex. It is difficult, if not impossible, to isolate sex and gender from the other intersections because feminism without race is not feminism (hooks, 2015) and feminism without intersectionality is likewise not feminism (Bilge and Collins, 2020). As Van Loon (2001) elucidates, women's lived experiences are very different from men's and are framed within patriarchy; not only is there a profound difference in my perceptions and my experiences but this occurs within a context whereby I have power, status and am encouraged to see only the dominant male privileged view. A participant asked me what right had I to look at (overwhelmingly) women's lives and how could I possibly understand them. The answer here is that by rights there is a slender justification; it is the altruistic aim of the well-intentioned ethnographer to acknowledge the weaknesses, the challenge of positionality and to be reflexive. That is, as here, to show enough detail for the reader to judge the robustness and validity of the research. I cannot walk in another's moccasins but in acknowledging this truth and by explicitly aiming to show my version of their voice is an ameliorative.

Of the differences in the experiences I have discussed in this chapter, age is well established in the ethnography literature and identified as the least difficult difference to bridge. Bilge and Collins (2020) repeatedly list age as last and least on their intersectionality analyses and as Harris and Patton (2019) indicate, gender, race, class and injustice-centred categories are the prime issues powering intersectionality. Islam, a religion appears omitted here but that is because it is racialised and included in the category of race, whereas age is left out because it is not seen as a fundamental category.

I am in my fifties, I have osteoarthritis, my energy levels and stamina do not compare well to the participants in their twenties. We have differing tastes in music, art, culture and speak different dialect of the same language. I set off from my house at 05:00 hours in the mornings and returned home as late as 22:00 hours, exhausted but still in need of writing and reflecting. Age was, thus, the final category of distance between us in terms of culture and physical energy. Hammersley and Atkinson (2007) make clear that the physicality of field work is demanding and that one must acknowledge this and pace oneself accordingly but as a practicality rather than a power or meaningful social disparity. As concerns culture, I am a student-centred engaging, interested humanist lecture and I have children of similar ages to the participants. I was and remain aware of the cultural generational differences and used sources for vocabulary and asked as we went. "Bare" meaning very, "butters" for unattractive are examples of the young Multicultural London English (MLE) that I now speak reasonably well (BBC R4, 2018). If I have heard of the genre of music that twenty-year-olds like then they have already ceased to like it and moved on.

Conclusions

In conclusion, this chapter has looked at one aspect of how a researcher may rationalise the validity of using ethnography to tell others' stories. Positionality is necessary to do this and it requires reflexivity; a looking at oneself in relation to others and the other that constitutes society. How this process effects the research in terms of collecting, validating, theme-finding, analysing and presenting the data is a necessary ongoing procedure. Intersectional theory offers a check list of categories of varying importance that require not simply ticking off in shopping list fashion but engaging with and interlinking. This chapter has looked at faith/religion, diet, race/ethnicity, social class, sex and gender, finally age as the intersectional categories needing inclusion. To address these, I had to show who I am, why I am researching this topic, what each category means and how each interacts with each other, with self-disclosure, insider/outsider ideas and me.

Fieldwork and ethnographic interviews have enabled me to show what I believe I have seen and what I perceive it to have meant. For example, I saw an event, noted it, reflected upon it and then fed back to the participants and their peers what I, an outsider, perceived I had witnessed. Where I perceived racism, Islamophobia and gender-based oppression it was sometimes identified back to me as something they experienced everyday and saw as unremarkable and "normal." The ensuing discussions between me and among the Muslim women themselves refined what I had seen and involved them offering clarity of meaning and brought a shared meaning closer, while accommodating differences. Reflexivity and positionality discussions are processes rather than end points and ones which contributed to the validity of the project.

A white Christian man undertaking a research project on Islamophobia must necessarily be reflexive on his positionality and I hope that this chapter has offered an adequate exposition of this complex but achievable requirement.

References

Ademolu, E. (2023) 'Birds of a feather (don't always) flock together: critical reflexivity of "outsiderness" as an "insider" doing qualitative research with one's "own people"', *Qualitative Research*, pp. 1–23. Available at: https://doi.org/10.1177/14687941221149596

Alejandro, A. (2021, January–December) 'How to problematise categories: building the methodological toolbox for linguistic reflexivity', *International Journal of Qualitative Methods*, 20, pp. 1–12. Available at: https://doi.org/10.1177/16094069211055572

Alejandro, A., & Zhao, L. (2023). Multi-method qualitative text and discourse analysis: a methodological framework. *Qualitative Inquiry*, 0(0). https://doi.org/10.1177/10778004231184421

All Party Parliamentary Group on British Muslims. (2018) *Islamophobia defined: the inquiry into a working definition of Islamophobia*. London: HMSO. Available at:

https://static1.squarespace.com/static/599c3d2febbd1a90cffdd8a9/t/5bfd1ea3352f5
31a6170ceee/1543315109493/Islamophobia+Defined.pdf (Accessed: 6 April 2023).

Anderson, E. (2022) *Black in white space: the enduring impact of color in everyday life*. London: The University of Chicago Press.

Bell, D. (1992) *Faces at the bottom of the well: the permanence of racism*. New York: Basic Books.

Bhatti, T. (2021) *Defining Islamophobia: a contemporary understanding of how expressions of Muslimness are targeted*. Muslim Council of Great Britain. Available at: https://mcb.org.uk/wp-content/uploads/2022/11/FULL-SPREAD-IslamophobiaReport_020321_compressed.pdf (Accessed: 6 April 2023).

Bonilla-Silva, E. (2021) *Racism without racists: color-blind racism and the persistence of racial inequality in America*. 6th edn. London: Rowman and Littlefield.

Bourdieu, P. (1977) *Outline to a Theory of Practice*. Cambridge: Cambridge University Press.

Braun, V. and Clarke, V. (2021) *Thematic analysis: a practical guide*. United Kingdom: London: SAGE Publications.

Braun, V. and Clarke, V. (2022) *Thematic analysis: a practical guide*. London: Sage.

Clarke, S and Garner, S. (2010) *White identities: a critical sociological approach*. London: Pluto Press.

Clifford, J. (1986) 'Introduction: partial truths,' in J. Clifford and G. E. Marcus (eds) *Writing culture: the poetics and politics of ethnography*. Berkeley: University of California Press, pp. 1–26.

Coffey, A. (1999) *The ethnographic self: fieldwork and the representation of identity*. London: Sage.

Collins, P. H. (2015) 'Intersectionality's definitional demands', *Annual Review of Sociology*, 41, pp. 1–20. Available at https://www.annualreviews.org/doi/10.1146/annurev-soc-073014-112142

Collins, P. H. and Bilge, S. (2016) *Intersectionality*. Cambridge: Polity Press.

Collins, P. H. and Bilge, S. (2020) *Intersectionality*. 2nd edn. Oxford: Wiley. ISBN: 978-1-509-53967-3

Coser, L. A. (1975) 'Merton's use of the European sociological condition', in L. A. Coser (ed) *The idea of social structure: papers in honor of Robert K. Merton*. New York: Harcourt Brace Jovanovich, pp. 85–102.

Crenshaw, K. W. (1989) 'Demarginalizing the intersection of race and sex: a Black feminist critique of antidiscrimination doctrine, feminist theory and antiracist politics', *University of Chicago Legal Forum*, (1), pp. 138–167.

Crenshaw, K. W. (1995) 'Mapping the margins: intersectionality, politics, and violence against women of color', in K. Crenshaw, N. Gotanda, G. Pellar, and K. Thomas (eds) *Critical race theory: the key writings that formed the movement*. New York: The New Press, pp. 357–383.

DiAngelo, R. J. (2019) *White fragility: why it's so hard for white people to talk about racism*. Boston, MA: Beacon Press.

Eddo-Lodge, R. (2017) *Why I'm no longer talking to white people about race*. London: Bloomsbury Circus.

Fleming, C. M. (2019) *How to be less stupid about race: on racism, white supremacy, and the racial divide: the essential guide to confronting white supremacy*. London: Beacon Press.

Folkes, L. (2022) 'Moving beyond "shopping list" positionality: using kitchen table reflexivity and in/visible tools to develop reflexive qualitative research', *Qualitative Research*, pp. 1–18. Available at: https://doi-org/10.1177/14687941221098922

Foreign, Commonwealth and Development Office. (2022) *International ministerial conference on freedom of religion or belief: London.* Available at: https://www.gov. uk/government/topical-events/international-ministerial-conference-on-freedom-of-religion-or-belief-london-2022 (Accessed: 5 March 2023).

Garner, S. (2007) *Racisms: an introduction.* London: Sage.

Geertz, C. (1973) *The Interpretation of Cultures.* New York: Basic Books.

Gholami, R. (2021) 'Critical race theory and Islamophobia: a challenging inequity in higher education', *Race, Ethnicity and Education,* 24(3), pp. 319–337. Available at: https://www.tandfonline.com/doi/full/10.1080/13613324.2021.1879770

Giddens, A. and Sutton, P. W. (2021) *Sociology.* 9th edn. Cambridge: Polity Press.

Gillborn, D. (2015) 'Intersectionality, critical race theory, and the primacy of racism: race, class, gender, and disability in education', *Qualitative Inquiry,* 21(3), pp. 277–287. Available at: https://doi.org/10.1177/1077800414557827

Goffman, E. (1959) *The presentation of self in everyday life.* London: Penguin.

Goffman, E. (1963) *Stigma: notes on the management of spoiled identity.* London: Penguin.

Goldberg, D. T. (2023) *The war on critical race theory or, the remaking of racism.* Cambridge: Polity Press.

Gray, D. E. (2014) *Doing research in the real world.* London: Sage.

Hall, S. (2021) 'Gramsci's relevance for the study of race and ethnicity', in P. Gilroy and R. W. Gilmore (compliers and editors), *Selected writings on race and difference.* Durham: Duke University Press, pp. 295–328.

Hammersley, M. and Atkinson, P. (2007) *Ethnography: principles in practice.* 3rd edn. London: Routledge.

Haraway, D. J. (1991) *Simians, cyborgs and women: the reinvention of nature.* Oxon: Routledge.

Harris, J and Patton, L (2019) 'Un/Doing Intersectionality through Higher Education Research', *Journal of Higher Education,* 90(3), pp. 347–372.

Hunt, J. C. (1989) *Psychoanalytic aspects of fieldwork.* London: Sage.

Jackson, M. (1989) *Paths towards a clearing: radical empiricism and ethnographic inquiry.* Bloomington and Indianapolis: Indiana University Press.

Kaufmann, E. and Harris, G. (2015) '"White flight" or positive contact? Local diversity and attitudes to immigration in Britain', *Comparative Political Studies,* 48(12), pp. 1563–1590. Available at: https://doi-org.ezproxy.mdx.ac.uk/10.1177/0010414015581684

Kleinman, S. and Copp, M. A. (1993) *Emotions and fieldwork.* Newbury Park: Sage Publications.

Kumar, D. (2021) *Islamophobia and the politics of empire.* 2nd edn. London: Verso.

Lentin, A. (2020) *Why race still matters.* Cambridge: Polity Press.

MacPherson, W. (1999) *The Stephen Lawrence inquiry.* Available at: https://assets. publishing.service.gov.uk/government/uploads/system/uploads/attachment_data/file/277111/4262.pdf (Accessed: 6 April 2023).

Marcus, G.E. and Mischer, M. (1999) *Anthropology as cultural critique: an experimental moment in the human sciences.* Chicago: University of Chicago Press.

Malik, A. and Wykes, E. (2018) *British Muslims in UK Higher Education Socio-political, religious and policy consideration.* London: The Bridge Institute for Research Policy.

Marcus, G. E. (1986) 'Contemporary problems of ethnography in the modern world system,' in J. Clifford and G. E. Marcus (eds) *Writing culture: the poetics and politics of ethnography.* Berkeley: University of California Press, pp. 165–193.

McCall, L. (2005) 'The complexity of intersectionality', *The University of Chicago Press Journals*, 30(3), pp. 1771–1800. Available at: http://www.jstor.org/stable/10.1086/426800 (Accessed: 12 January 2018).

Ministry of Justice. (2022) *Diversity of the judiciary: legal professions, new appointments and current post-holders – 2022 statistics.* Available at: https://www.gov.uk/government/statistics/diversity-of-the-judiciary-2022-statistics/diversity-of-the-judiciary-legal-professions-new-appointments-and-current-post-holders-2022-statistics (Accessed: 6 April 2023).

Mir, S. (2014) *Muslim American women on campus: undergraduate social life and identity.* Chapel Hill: The University of North Carolina Press.

Moosavi, L. (2014) 'The racialization of Muslim converts in Britain and their experiences of Islamophobia', *Critical Sociology*, 41(1), pp. 41–56.

Morrison, T. (2017) *The origin of others.* London: Harvard University Press.

Morrison, T. (2019) *Mouth full of blood: essays, speeches, meditations.* London: Chatto and Windus.

'Multicultural English.' (2018) *Word of mouth.* BBC Radio 4, 2 October. Available at: https://www.bbc.co.uk/sounds/play/m0000mk0 (Accessed: 3 April 2023).

Munby, J. (2013) 'The courts are secular, says top family judge'. Interview with Sir James Munby. Interviewed by C. Baksi for *The Law Society Gazette*, 29 October. Available at: https://www.lawgazette.co.uk/law/the-courts-are-secular-says-top-family-judge/5038456.article#:~:text=The%20law%20has%20a%20neutral,nature%20of%20the%20judges'%20job (Accessed: 25 January 2023).

Najib, K. (2022) *Spatialized Islamophobia.* Abingdon: Routledge.

Nursing and Midwifery Council. (2018) *The code: professional standards of practice and behaviour for nurses, midwives and nursing associates.* Available at: https://www.nmc.org.uk/standards/code/ (Accessed: 20 March 2023).

Office for National Statistics. (2022) *The national statistics socio-economic classification (NS-SEC).* Available at: https://www.ons.gov.uk/methodology/classificationsandstandards/otherclassifications/thenationalstatisticssocioeconomicclassificationnssecrebasedonsoc2010 (Accessed: 5 January 2023).

Paradis, E. and Sutkin, G. (2016) 'Beyond a good story: from Hawthorne effect to reactivity in health professions education research', *Medical Education*, 51(1), pp. 31–39. Available at: https://doi.org/10.1111/medu.13122

Pillow, W. (2003) 'Confessions, catharsis, or cure? Rethinking the uses of reflexivity as methodological power in qualitative research', *International Journal of Qualitative Studies in Education,* 16(2), pp. 175–196. Available at: https://doi.org/10.1080/0951839032000060635.

Reyes, V. (2020) 'Ethnographic toolkit: strategic positionality and researchers' visible and invisible tools in field research', *Ethnography*, 21(2), pp. 220–240. Available at: https://doi.org/10.1177/1466138118805121

Riessman, K. C. (2007) *Narrative methods for the human science.* London: Sage.

Rock, P. (2001) 'Symbolic interactionism and ethnography,' in P. Atkinson, A. Coffey, S. Delamont, J. Lofland and L. Lofland (eds), *Handbook of ethnography.* London: Sage, pp. 26–38.

Rollock, N. (2022) *The racial code: tales of resistance and survival.* Milton Keynes: Allen Lane.

Rossiter, M. W. (1993) 'The Matthew Matilda effect in science', *Social Studies of Science,* 23, pp. 325–341. Available at: https://doi/pdf/10.1177/030631293023002004

Runneymede. (1997) *Islamophobia: a challenge for us all.* Available at: https://www.
runnymedetrust.org/publications/islamophobia-a-challenge-for-us-all (Accessed:
5 January 2023).

Runneymede. (2016) *Islamophobia – 20 years on, still a challenge for us all.* Available at: https://www.runnymedetrust.org/blog/islamophobia-20-years-on-still-a-
challenge-for-us-all (Accessed: 20 January 2020).

Said, E. W. (1978) *Orientalism.* Harmondsworth: Penguin.

Spradley, J. P. (1975) *Participant observation.* Long Grove, IL: Waveland Press, Inc.

Spradley, J. P. (1979) *The ethnographic interview.* Long Grove, IL: Waveland Press, Inc.

Sue, D. W. (2015) *Race talk and the conspiracy of silence.* Hoboken, NJ: John Wiley
& Sons.

Van Loon, J. (2001) 'Ethnography: a critical turn in cultural studies', in P. Atkinson,
A. Coffey, S. Delamont, J. Lofland and L. Lofland (eds), *Handbook of ethnography.* London: Sage, pp. 273–284.

Varisco, D. M. (2005) *Islam obscured: the rhetoric of anthropological representation.*
New York: Palgrave Macmillan.

Vindrola-Padros, C. (2021) *Rapid ethnographies: a practical guide.* Cambridge: Cambridge University Press.

6 The Nursing and Midwifery Council's (NMC) role in integrating internationally educated nurses (IENs) in the UK health care

Iyore Monday Ugiagbe

In this chapter I discuss the role of the UK statutory nurse registration body, the Nursing and Midwifery Council (NMC), in integrating internationally educated nurses (IENs) into UK health care. Critical race theory (CRT), post-colonial theory (PCT) and intersectionality theory (IT) were used in my PhD to employ to critique existing nurse registration structures, processes and practices in UK health care and existing immigration policies and procedures regarding IENs' recruitment, retention and integration. I argue that the NMC has contributed to the continuity of nurse shortages in the UK and persisting discrimination in UK health care. I draw on my experiences in the NHS in different roles and capacities and on interviews undertaken as part of my PhD, which explored the lived experiences of nurses of Nigerian heritage on their integration into UK health care post-NMC registration. I discuss the NMC's role in addressing nurse shortages in the UK since the inception of nurse regulation in 1919. I link the NMC's role in formulating policies on nurse training and recruitment with changing immigration policies since its creation and how it has overtly facilitated discrimination in nurse recruitment and retention in the UK. I discuss the impact of the NMC's policies on immigration and integration on the lived experiences of nurses as they adapt to life and work in the UK.

The use of reflexivity in my PhD study richly influences this chapter. Reflexivity is '...*the process of a continual internal dialogue and critical self-evaluation of researcher's positionality as well as active acknowledgement and explicit recognition that this position may affect the research process and outcome*' (Berger, 2015: 220). Reflexivity enables the elucidation of positionality and how formulating views concerning individuals' values, interests and beliefs may impact the research objectives (Cousin, 2009; cited in Ugiagbe, 2022). I have used my reflective journal as a valuable and positive means for constructing knowledge (Brydon-Miller and Coghlan, 2014, cited in Ugiagbe, 2022) and as a tool to encourage my reflexivity (Mann, 2016). This allowed me to use my previous knowledge and understanding further to interpret (McConnell-Henry et al., 2009) the role of the NMC in integrating

DOI: 10.4324/9781003269915-6

IEN into the UK health care system. This chapter concludes that effectively integrating IENs is a significant ingredient for addressing nurse shortages and improving quality patient care in the UK health care system.

Recruitment of internationally educated nurses in the NHS

The establishment of the NHS and the effects of the Second World War contributed to the migration of several minority ethnic groups in the UK. On establishing the NHS in July 1948, there were 54,000 nurse vacancies, predominantly in the services for mental health, chronic illness and geriatric care (Batnitzky and McDowell, 2011). In the first four decades of the NHS, IENs were recruited for student nurse programmes and junior roles in UK health care (Snow and Jones, 2011) to fill these vacancies, and such nurses found it challenging to obtain a promotion in the NHS (Smith et al., 2006; Henry, 2007).

Nurses from the British colonies (now part of the Commonwealth of Nations) formed the bulk of migrant nurses recruited between the late 1940s and 1970s. The UK's ethnic landscape was drastically altered following the post-war migration in the 1940s, of Black African nurses into the NHS. Successive governments sought to allay public anxiety by introducing tighter controls around immigration (Snow and Jones, 2011). Migrant nurses were discriminated against as they were considered non-white and cultural outsiders (Batnitzky and McDowell, 2011). Following this period, racist immigration policies were propounded following the UK's admission to the European Union (EU) (Gentleman, 2022), and the UK 1971 Immigration Act curtailed IENs' recruitment from the Commonwealth (Snow and Jones, 2011) cited in Reynolds (2019).

The introduction of a new Nursing Associate programme on 26 July 2019 (NMC, 2020) and the continued recruitment of IENs using discriminatory policy guidelines on international recruitment (Ugiagbe et al., 2022) have not resolved the nurse shortage crisis in the UK. As of September 2019, the Royal College of Nursing (RCN) advised that the NHS was short of 40,000 nurses, increasing to 50,000 nursing vacancies in the UK by 2020 (RCN, 2019, 2020).

Consequently, it is fair to say that since the formation of the NHS, UK immigration policy has been shaped by the belief that internationally educated African-descent (black) nurses were needed in UK health care but were not 'wanted' in the UK. British immigration policy, Spencer (1997) argues, has operated in a way that makes it difficult for African-descent (black) nurses to settle in the United Kingdom. However, it has taken until 2020 for racial discrimination to be openly discussed as a significant issue in UK nursing because a persistent colour-blind approach, which is race and ethnicity neutral, has been the practice in the recruitment and integration of IENs (Hilario et al., 2017; Ugiagbe et al., 2022).

Role of the national registration body in internationally educated nurses' recruitment and integration: Pre- and post-NMC registration

In 1919 the UK government presented a bill to Parliament to establish a national nurse registration body, the General Nursing Council (GNC). The UK Nursing Register opened in September 1921, and Ethel Gordon Fenwick became the first nurse to join the register. The national nurse registration body is now the NMC. The NMC's primary purpose is to protect the public *'through maintaining a register of nurses, midwives and health visitors, setting and monitoring education standards through practice and conduct, and handling complaints about misconduct and unfitness to practise of those on the register'* (Thewlis, 2003: 1).

The NMC sets the standards of education, training, conduct and performance required of nurses and midwives in delivering patient care. A registered charity, the NMC is also accountable to Parliament, and the Professional Standards Authority oversees its functions for health and social care (NMC, 2020). Thus, the registration body has always been and continues to be subject directly or indirectly to influence from the UK government.

The NMC is the professional body responsible for validating and registering IENs to practice in the UK health care system. As Jayaweera (2015) argues, there has been a constant cycle of recruiting fluctuating numbers of IENs to fill the care gap in the UK health care system. This recruitment occurs in reaction to national health workforce shortages and is an essential and recurrent strategy in the UK nurse recruitment policy (RCN, 2003). However, there is no clearly defined process or procedure for maximising the long-term benefits, such as retaining internationally recruited nurses' post-NMC registration (Smith et al., 2006). This lack of strategy or policy questions the level of commitment of the various health care policy organisations to develop a sustainable solution to the issue of nurse shortage that has been problematic since the inception of the NHS.

According to Yu (2008), the adaptation process for IENs may be divided into a period of transition (initial adaptation) which is short term, and a period of integration (long-term adaptation). The NMC publishes competency standards required of newly registered nurses (NMC, 2018). Yu (2008) asserts that IENs become functionally competent in nursing duties and obtain their registration within the first year of recruitment. The nurse registration body has promoted and supported initial adaptation to engage the nurses in the clinical area. It has yet to publish standards for the long-term integration of international nurses into UK health care or define what integration might mean for IENs. The registration body and employers appear to be concerned with programmes that will yield short-term immediate transitional needs so that IENs can be put to work as soon as practicable and maintain staffing levels in the care setting (Smith et al., 2006; Ugiagbe et al., 2022). The programmes are designed to help adapt or transition IENs into the workplace. There is a need for more interest in the benefits of integration in the wider lived experiences of IENs, their integration into British society and the settlement of families (Ugiagbe, 2022). This lack of interest has contributed to the continued shortage of registered nurses in the UK health care sector as IENs fail to be promoted to their full abilities and suggests that the NHS discriminates against non-white nurses (Smith et al., 2006; Allan and Westwood, 2016). It has done this partly through the historical and contemporary discriminatory regulation of IENs by the NMC. The NMC has effectively worked in alignment with the British government to allay public anxiety by introducing tighter controls around registering IENs since the establishment of the NHS.

This pattern of systemic discrimination may be seen in the historical overview of NMC regulation in Table 6.1, which summarises significant NMC policy changes on IEN. I have divided NMC regulation into five historical periods and the current period: 1948–the 1980s, the 1980s–2000, 2000–2007, 2007–2016 and 2016–2022, post-2022. The data in this table forms the basis of the discussion of the racist migration policies and NMC regulation of IENs' registration in the next section.

It can be seen from Table 6.1 that over seven decades, it has become progressively more challenging for IENs to come to work in the UK both in terms

Table 6.1 Summary of requirements since the establishment of the NHS

1948–1980s	• The nurse registration body was the General Nursing Council (GNC), later the United Kingdom Central Council for Nursing Midwifery and Health Visiting (UKCC). • Nurses recruited to UK health care directly from Commonwealth countries • Nurses' education in the Commonwealth was comparable to UK training • Nurses from the British colonies (now part of the Commonwealth of Nations) formed the bulk of migrant nurses recruited between the late 1940s and the late 1970s, facilitated by the 1919 Nurses Act. • The 1919 Nurses Act meant that nurses who trained outside of the UK in any of the British empires were eligible to be on the register and could practice in the UK. • The Nurses' Act of 1949 widened the definition of 'nurse' and relaxed criteria that dictated who was eligible to practise in the UK. • Recruitment from overseas in the 1960s and 1970s continued as part of government policy to solve labour shortages in Britain • No official centralised test of the English language or clinical competence test for nurses recruited from the Commonwealth • No official period of supervised practice for recruited IENs • The UK 1971 Immigration Act curtailed IEN recruitment from the Commonwealth

(Continued)

Table 6.1 (Continued)

1980s–2000	• New laws were introduced post-1971, and work permits for IENs were abolished in 1983 • Nurse registration body (UKCC; later NMC) determines specific requirements about the length of clinical placements for each IEN applicant • Average length of clinical placement for nurses trained in Commonwealth countries was between 3 and 6 months. • Supervised practice/Adaptation programme in UK health care settings evolved for IENs. • No official, centralised test of the English language or competence test is required of IENs.
2000–2007	• Relaxation of the work permit system in 1999 to enable the realisation of the NHS plan to recruit additional nurses. • NMC determines specific requirements for the length of clinical placements for IENs. • Average length of clinical placements for supervised practice is likely to be between 3 and 6 months. • A period of supervised practice for IENs in approved health care settings by the NMC is introduced. • Overseas Nurse Programme (ONP); renamed Supervised Practice Programme, is introduced in approved Higher Education Institutions (HEI) for every applicant trained outside the EEA (European Economic Area) • The Return to Nursing Programme was introduced in approved HEI for nurses not in practice for three years or more wishing to return to practice. • No official, centralised test of the English language or competence test for IENs. • Employers are to give ORN appropriate support to improve IENs' language skills through the transition into working in the UK (NHS Employers, 2017a, 2017b).
2007–2016	• Nursing removed from the Home Office Shortage of Occupations list in 2007 • The Immigration Acts of 2014 and 2016 introduced the 'hostile environment' policy, which later changed to a 'compliant environment'. • IENs must complete the International English Language Testing System (IELTS) or the Occupational English Test (OET). • Test results must not be over two years old when submitting the registration application. • At the time of the application, the applicant must have practised as a registered nurse or midwife for at least 12 months (full-time or part-time). After qualifying applicants have been trained for longer than this, they must have practised for at least 450 hours in the previous three years. • Applicants must hold a current registration or licence without restriction with the licensing authority or registration body in the country where they qualified or have been practising.

(Continued)

Table 6.1 (Continued)

	• Applicants must have completed at least ten years of school education before starting a post-secondary education nursing or midwifery training programme. This will lead to registration as an entry-level registered nurse or midwife in their home country. • Official centralised test of competence introduced for IENs. Part one of the test is a multiple-choice examination, and part two is a practical examination called an OSCE (objective structured clinical examination). • Employers are responsible for support to the IEN to improve their language skills (NHS Employers, 2017a, 2017b). • Nursing was reinstated in the shortage of Occupations list in 2015 due to the continued lack of nurses.
2016–2022	• Effective 28/06/16, internationally educated nurses: • Must complete the International English Language Testing System (IELTS) or the Occupational English Test (OET). • A minimum score of seven overall and in each of the four skills in not more than two sittings in IELTS. • Both IELTS tests must be within six months, and no score must be below 6.5 in any of the areas across both tests. • Exempted from writing IELTS or OET where a candidate has registration and one year's practise with a nursing or midwifery regulator in a country where English is the first and native language, and a language assessment was required for registration. • It is the employers' responsibility to support IEN) to improve their language skills (NHS Employers, 2017a, 2017b).
2023–	• New test combining rules introduced. IENs must achieve the required scores in all four domains across two tests. • Scores can now be combined across two test sittings taken up to 12 months apart, rather than the previous six-month limit. • The minimum scores are now standardised to allow the combination of test scores if an applicant misses one of the required scores by 0.5 (IELTS) or half a grade (OET) with another test of the same type to meet requirements. • The minimum writing score now changed to 6.0 (IELTS) or C/250–290 (OET). However, IEN must score at least 6.5 (IELTS) or C+/300–340 (OET) in writing in the second test sitting to combine this score. • Employers can submit supporting information for applicants trained in English in a country where English is not a majority-spoken language and are working in an unregulated role in UK health and social care. • IEN must have worked in a health and care setting for at least one year. • Evidence is required that their training and assessment were in English.

of testing by the NMC and employers and in terms of available support when adapting to life in the UK. In the face of accusations of structural and institutional discrimination (Ugiagbe et al., 2022), the NMC (2023) published some changes to language requirements. Applicants can now combine test results and IENs, whose training was in English in a country where English is not a majority-spoken language and are working in an unregulated role in UK health and social care, can now show evidence that their nurse training and assessment were in English. Consequently, through their employers, they will now be exempt from sitting the compulsory English language competence examination (NMC, 2023). However, it is now compulsory that the IEN must have worked in a health and care setting for at least one year as a health care support worker (NMC, 2023) as one of the requirements for the IEN to be considered suitable for commencing registration with the NMC. This last requirement is evidence of further oppression by the NMC of marginalised racial groups who comprise the vast majority of migrant nurses to the UK (Allan and Westwood, 2016). The marginalisation that the NMC processes result in is influenced by the micro-politics of power and macro-dynamics from historical and structural perspectives (Kirkham and Anderson, 2002: 2:2).

Racist migration policies and NMC regulation of internationally educated nurses' registration

The 1919 Nurses Act meant that nurses who trained outside of the UK in any British colonies were eligible to be included in the UK register and could practice in the UK (see Table 6.1) as they were subjects of the British Empire and held the same rights as British born subjects – known as 'Civis Brittanicus sum' (I am a British citizen). From the 1940s to the 1950s, the UK government managed the recruitment drive so that untrained overseas nurses were recruited as student nurses to staff British hospitals. More registered nurses left the UK than overseas-trained nurses than came to the UK as white UK nurses left the UK to staff the British colonial hospitals in the British Empire, usually as Chief Nursing Officers and other senior posts (Spencer, 1997). The 1943 Nurses' Act entrenched the register of assistant nurses, or State Enrolled Assistant Nurses (SEAN). The introduction of this enrolled nurse cadre, Solano and Rafferty (2007) argue, marked the start of the division of the nursing workforce between the state registered nurse (SRN), the state enrolled nurse (EN) and the unregistered Health Care Assistants (HCA), or Auxiliary Nurses. This division was based on discrimination and racism that has structured the nursing workforce to the present day. It widened access for recruiting candidates from the colonies to training positions in the UK, but British-born (white) nurses dominated education programmes leading to registration and nursing leadership and education positions. The UKCC (now NMC) '*declared an end to the enrolled nurse training programme and promised that all enrolled nurses could, if they wished, convert to the first level of the nursing register*' (Webb, 2000: 119). In other words, introducing SEAN failed and had no merit in addressing the nurse recruitment and shortage problems in the UK health care system. The introduction of the SEAN '*Instilled the professional hierarchy that was to favour British registered nurses, but it also impacted on professional culture, reinforcing assumptions based on race, class and social background*' (Solano and Rafferty, 2007: 5).

The NMC's philosophy and practice have not altered today. It is open to question why following the restructuring of nurse education to graduate-only (Peate and Lane, 2017), many of the nurses (SENs) who were judged previously as lacking the cognitive abilities and motivation to train to become qualified SRNs (Snow and Jones, 2011) were then accepted in UK Universities to undergo the conversion course to be registered nurses. It suggests another quick-fix measure to change policy and practice when the regulatory body deems it fit to ameliorate the shortage of registered nurses in the UK health care system.

The Nurses' Act of 1949 facilitated the GNC to alter *'the definition of 'nurse', and relaxing criteria that dictated who was eligible to practice in the UK'* (Solano and Rafferty, 2007: 5). The change and relaxation of criteria were necessary to enable many more candidates from the colonies to join the nurse register to help deal with the nurse shortage in the UK. This requirement also led to the government's relaxation of immigration control from the 1950s until the 1970s (Snow and Jones, 2011). During this period (1948–the 1970s – see Table 6.1), overseas nurses were recruited to the UK health care system directly from Commonwealth countries; their education in the Commonwealth was seen as comparable to UK training, and there was no official, centralised test of English language required of IENs from the commonwealth countries. There was no official competence test for nurses recruited from the Commonwealth, or an official period of supervised practice or adaptation for recruited overseas nurses from the colonies. The IENs' English language competence or standard of nursing practice was not considered sub-standard during this period. However, in the present era, these same IENs (or their descendants!) are judged unfit for registration by the NMC without succeeding in compulsory objective structured clinical examination (OSCE) competence tests and satisfactory evidence through employers to show that nurse training and assessment were in English to become NMC registered nurses (NMC, 2023).

In line with the Conservative government policy of the 1980s that abolished the work permit system for IENs (see Table 6.1), the nurse registration body (UKCC; later NMC) introduced specific requirements regarding the length of clinical placements for each IEN applicant. The average length of clinical placement for nurses trained in Commonwealth countries was likely to be between three and six months. The IEN was required to have a non-salaried supervised practice/adaptation programme in several UK health care settings. During this period, no official English language or competencies-based tests was needed from IEN nurses. The dramatic change from the automatic recognition and registration of Commonwealth nurses by the GNC to the requirement for a period of supervised practice/adaptation introduced by the UKCC was influenced by protectionism in UK politics at the time, which resulted in increased calls for reduced immigration amidst waves of anti-migrant rhetoric and feeling (Reynolds, 2019; Ugiagbe et al., 2022).

During the 1990s, there was a rise in the number of nurses leaving the register and a steady decrease in the number of nurses joining. The acute shortage of nurses arising from protectionist immigration policies of the Conservative governments of the 1980s led to the Labour government's relaxation of the work permit system in 1999 to enable the realisation of the NHS Plan (DOH, 2000), which aimed to recruit thousands of IENs. The UKCC was renamed the NMC in April 2002 under the same government (1999–2007). At this time, the NMC still determined the specific requirements concerning the length of clinical placements. The average clinical placement for supervised practice was three to six months in approved health care settings. The NMC introduced the Overseas Nurse Programme (ONP), renamed Supervised Practice Programme (SPP), in approved Higher Education Institutes for every applicant trained outside the EEA (European Economic Area). It also introduced the Return to Nursing Programme for nurses with NMC registration who may have left nursing in the UK but now wish to return to practice. During this period of ONP or SPP, there were still no official, centralised tests for IEN on English language competence or clinical skills competencies. As a result of the political will to increase the number of nurses, this period (2001–2004) witnessed the highest number of IENs registering with the NMC (Buchan, 2007). The number of IENs was more than nurses trained in UK institutions. This situation led to further calls for immigration controls to tighten the conditions required for IEN nurses to register in the UK (Reynolds, 2019).

From April 2005 to March 2006, the number of IEN registrants began to fall with the introduction of compulsory ONP or SPP by the NMC. By 2007, nursing was again removed from the shortage of occupations list, only temporarily reinstated in 2015 due to a continued lack of nurses (NHS, 2015). It is necessary to restate that the bulk of IENs seeking registration in the UK remain from previous British colonies and the Commonwealth of nation-states (Solano and Rafferty, 2007).

The IENs' English language competence or standard of nursing practice was not considered sub-standard from the inception of the NHS in 1948 until the sudden introduction of compulsory language competency in 2005. These IENs were recruited into a racist nursing workforce where efforts were made to assign nurses from the colonies to lower positions (SEAN) and training programmes rather than promote them to management and leadership roles in nursing (Smith et al., 2006). In line with successive governments' efforts to ease public anxiety by introducing tighter controls around immigration (Snow and Jones, 2011), IENs with African heritage are disproportionately represented in referrals to the NMC on allegations of poor communication issues. Still, they were more likely to have no case to answer. The crux of the matter was not about poor communication by the African heritage nurses. Instead, it concerns these nurses' poor integration by the employers and teamwork in the clinical environment (West and Nayar, 2019).

Testing of Internationally Educated Nurses

In 1884 Lord Rosebury used the phrase 'Commonwealth of Nations' to describe the new relationship between Britain and her colonies

> … autonomous Communities within the British Empire, equal in status, in no way subordinate one to another in any aspect of their domestic or external affairs, though united by a common allegiance to the Crown, and freely associated as members of the British Commonwealth of Nations.
>
> (Nexus, 2020: 1)

The UK has directly maintained ties with the colonies in neo-colonialism, actively maintaining bilateral relations with the old colonies, promoting socio-economic, educational, cultural and British political interests (Reynolds, 2019). The majority of the countries in the Commonwealth of Nations patterned their education and training after the education system in the UK during the colonial era. This led to the establishment in the late 20th century of the Commonwealth of Learning to encourage the development and sharing of open learning and distance education knowledge, resources and technology (Nexus Strategic Partnerships Limited, 2016). This directly contributed to the recruitment of nurses from the colonies from the 1940s to 1970s to work in the NHS.

The similarity in nurse education and training between the UK and ex-colonies (Smith et al., 2006) made non-EU (from the Commonwealth) trained nurses fit to practice nursing in the UK from the 1940s to 1970s and to be accepted into pre-registration education programmes. However, the reaction to IEN nurses in the UK changed over time, as shown in Table 6.1, as immigration controls tightened generally and the NMC increased its requirements for IEN to show themselves fit for practice in the UK (Smith et al., 2006). In a study by Smith et al. (2006) on Equal Opportunities for IEN and Other health care Professionals (REOH), the authors found that UK health care managers had begun to require better preparation before employing or promoting IENs. Smith et al. showed that highly educated non-EU nurses who were fluent in English, and competent were not being promoted on rather flimsy grounds. If we compare medical staff and nurses, it is puzzling that the UK government has encouraged recruitment of medical doctors from some Commonwealth countries, such as India (Snow and Jones, 2011) but has yet to do the same consistently for nurses from these countries. Yet there are similarities in medical and nursing curricula and historical connections between educational institutions, colleges and personnel in the Commonwealth and the UK. Despite the similarity in nurse education and training between the UK and ex-colonies (Smith et al., 2006), a compulsory clinical competence and English language test were introduced for migrant nurses wishing to register and practice in the United Kingdom in 2005 (NMC, 2017a). It is unclear why the NMC disregarded qualities that had been satisfactory up to the 1970s and chose to subject this group of non-EU nurses from the ex-colonies to compulsory tests in English. This policy change has been described as a restrictive and discriminatory practice (Likupe, 2006; Ugiagbe et al., 2022). It seems that the NMC has been subject in its regulatory systems to imposing unstated, discriminatory conditions which determine the suitability of IENs to practice in the UK. These conditions are unrelated to clinical ability, knowledge and competence and, therefore, racist. The NMC tests of suitability in language and competencies contribute to reducing migration to the UK and assuring the public that IENs and midwives are capable of safe and effective practice (Likupe, 2006) without evidence that practice before the tests was unsafe.

A compulsory English language test was introduced to the United Kingdom in 2005 (NMC, 2017a). In 2016, the NMC extended the IELTS requirement to nurses within the EU/EEA (NMC, 2017b; RCN, 2017). This has led to discriminatory and racist practices as IENs who do not pass their language tests are employed by NHS trusts and work as health care support workers until they pass the test (Allan and Westwood, 2016). Each test is expensive for nurses from developing countries because of the exorbitant exchange rates. For example, the alternative test, the Occupational English Test (OET), costs £340 and is higher than the price of IELTS (£150–£200), the computer-based test (CBT) for IENs to work in the UK costs £83 (Takeielts. britishcouncil.org, 2018; NMC, 2019), and all parts of the test need to be passed simultaneously, which has led to some IENs resitting the language tests multiple times (Allan and Westwood, 2016; Ugiagbe et al., 2022). The NMC's position on assessing IENs for registration and practice in the UK and the rule of employing IENs as Health care Assistants if they fail their language test seems to enhance institutionalised racial and ethnic disadvantages in the NHS (Smith et al., 2006; Allan and Westwood, 2016) and will continue to promote '*recruiting BME communities to the less desirable, low paid "BBC" (British Bottom Care) [jobs]*' (MacGregor 2007 cited in Allan and Westwood, 2015: 3). As stated previously, due to the Labour government's political will to increase the number of registered nurses in the NHS, the NMC promoted an IENs registration policy that made it possible for the highest number of IENs registered in the UK between 2001 and 2004. To protect the domestic job market for student nurses, the NMC introduced a new policy from April 2005 to March 2006, and the number of IENs began to fall with the introduction of compulsory ONP by the NMC. The government further tightened the immigration requirement by removing nursing from the shortage of occupations list. The NMC policy and the government immigration changes resulted in a severe lack of registered nurses in the UK. The government was forced to reinstate nursing on the shortage of Occupations list in 2015.

'The Hand of Esau but the Voice of Jacob'

According to a former Chief Nursing Officer (CNO),

> ... nursing has evolved and advanced over the years. This will continue to grow. Changing demographics means that more nurses will start their careers in community, primary care or public health roles; they will work in voluntary or the independent sector and in integrated teams with social care, educators and others.
>
> (Cummings, 2014: 2)

This being the case, it is difficult to see how the shift in the NMC position from an SSP or the Overseas Nurses Programme to assessment via online testing for non-EU/EEA trained nurses may be used to meet the evolving role of the UK nurse in the 21st century and help address the constant shortage of registered nurses in the UK. This is even more difficult to understand when consideration is given to the fact that some integration built into the Supervised Practice Nurses Programme was non-existent in the current method of non-EU nurses gaining registration.

In the first 57 years of the NHS (1948 until 2005), there was no compulsory test in English or OSCE for nurses from commonwealth countries. In the last 15–20 years (2005–2022), stringent measures have been introduced to prevent migrant nurses from joining the NMC register. This is a puzzling development when there is an increasing shortage of registered nurses in the NHS and a policy agreement of the government for international nurse recruitment to tackle the persistent chronic nurse shortage in the UK. It is expedient to query why nurses from Anglophone countries are grouped with other nurses from other parts of the world whose training is not conducted in English or subjected to compulsory English and clinical skills tests. On paper, an employer must ensure that the IEN is given the appropriate support to improve their language skills through the transition into working in the UK (NHS Employers, 2017a, 2017b). However, this has not been the focus of practice or supported in the literature. The rationale for this may be that the NMC has focussed attention not on integrating IENs into UK health care but on streamlining the registration of migrant nurses in indirect support of the immigration policies of successive governments and promoting the confidence of the populace in the practice of international nurses.

The nursing register opened in September 1921 for nurses of good character (Shepherd, 2019). The standard required to be admitted to the register by the GNC was that aspiring nurses had to be aged 21 or over, able to give three references of good character, and able to demonstrate they had at least one year's training and two years' subsequent practice. The council also decided on disciplinary procedures (Shepherd, 2019: 9). However, these processes were not value-free. In discussing nursing and colonialism, Rafferty and Solano (2007: 148, 153) state that there is a lack of research into the relationship between nursing and the empire and little attention focused on the administrative and policy links between formal government involvement and international nurse recruitment (148), and argue further that there is a need to acknowledge the degree to which professional registration body has colluded and benefited from international recruitment in the expansion of their own professional 'empire' (153). The UK government has, since the establishment of the nurse registration body, attempted to extricate its link with the nurse registration body; for example, in 1919, the Colonial Nursing Association (CNA) changed its name to Overseas Nursing Service (ONS) to redefine itself outside the discourse of colonialism (Rafferty and Solano, 2007).

As previously stated, in July 1948, there were 54,000 nurse vacancies in NHS, predominantly in mental health, chronic sick and geriatric care (Batnitzky and McDowell, 2011). As of September 2019, UK health care was short of 40,000 nurses, increasing to 50,000 nursing vacancies in the NHS in the UK by 2020 (RCN, 2019, 2020). Despite this shortage, the NHS continues to function and is often rated among the best health care systems in the world. I argue here that it is through the exploitation of the overworked, understaffed and underpaid nurses including IENs, that the system continues to function. The central political and economic philosophy facilitated by the government to recruit nurses from the colonies between 1948 and the 1970s is the guide in tackling the nurse shortage and formulating nurse recruitment policies in the 21st century. International nurse recruitment in the 1960s and 1970s continued as part of government policy to solve Britain's labour shortages (Beishon et al., 1995 cited in Likupe, 2006), and this international recruitment is an essential and recurrent strategy in the UK nurse recruitment policy in the 21st century (RCN, 2003). Health Minister Enoch Powell, who was to later give the infamous 'Rivers of Blood Speech' on 20 April 1968, championed the recruitment of IENs in the early 1960s. The policy executed by Enoch Powell was to ensure that 'the *British colonies and former colonies provided a constant supply of cheap labour to meet staffing shortages in the NHS*' (Snow and Jones, 2011:2). And as a result, some 3000–5000 Jamaican nurses worked in British hospitals by 1965, and 10,566 international student nurses from the colonies by 1972. By 1977 international nurse recruits represented 12% of Britain's student nurse and midwife population (Snow and Jones, 2011: 2). In an innovative economic exploitative practice, the student nurses were regarded as employees of the hospital where the students had their training and were placed on low wages and included in workforce numbers. During the NHS's early decades, there was a widespread assumption that international nurses and nursing students would return to their home country after completing their nurse training or initial contract (Snow and Jones, 2011). This expectation turned out not to be the case because it was a politically and economically motivated expectation. Geddes (2003: 35) states that the UK immigration laws '*were based on the assumption that men were the breadwinners and women were dependants who would follow their husbands'*. Unfortunately, this assumption failed to consider the personal, economic and social development preferences or needs of the IENs. The majority of IENs are female (Geddes, 2003), and some of these nurses were perhaps in their late teens or early twenties and, therefore, may have started new relationships or families and may well have been led to make a recent decision to settle in the UK on a permanent or long term basis. The older nurses may have invited their spouses and children to join them in the UK. According to Kofman (1999), the UK lost its case to prevent male members from joining their female counterparts at the European Court of Human Rights (ECHR) because the UK law was discriminatory. The reaction of the UK Conservative government to this defeat at the ECHR was to introduce the 'primary purpose' rule in 1980. The Labour government abolished the 'primary purpose' rule in 1997 partly to enable the labour government to realise the NHS Plan (2000) to recruit over 10,000 nurses.

Due to racial prejudice, Spencer (1997) reports that though Prime Minister Atlee gave a public welcome to the African-descent (black) passengers aboard the Empire Windrush, *the British government, in a period of acute labour shortage, 'did not turn to its empire for additional labour'*. The discriminatory attitude and preference for European Volunteer Migrants (EVM) over African-descent (black) migrants by the UK government post-second world war was the reason behind the refusal to recruit more nurses from the Commonwealth despite the availability and willingness of nurses in the region populated by African-descent (black) nurses to join the UK nursing workforce (Solano and Rafferty, 2007). This covert preference appears to have motivated the NMC to introduce the conditions for IENs joining the register, for example, the introduction of requirements in the test of English language and clinical skills competency for nurses in former British colonies. Ugiagbe et al. (2022) see this practice as evidence of structural and institutional racism against international nurses from Anglophone African Countries. They argue that the NMC facilitates the establishment of the tests and normalises it in professional discourse.

According to Spencer (1997: 55), the *'attitude and approach to immigration taken by the Labour government of 1941–1955 had little difference in character from that of the Conservative successors'*. This understanding may mean a broad agreement to continue the discriminatory policy laid down by the Labour government led by PM Atlee and assiduously executed by PM Winston Churchill. It may also explain why Spencer (2011) stated in her book 'Migration Debate' that the *policy paradigm had its origins in the post-war era and has not adjusted to the migration patterns of modern times'* (p.201). The immigration policy in practice from 1945 to 1955 exposes 'the myth of Civis Britannicus sum' because *'the British immigration policy operated in a way that was intended to make it difficult for Asian and Black British subjects to settle in the United Kingdom* (Spencer,1997: 21).

Thus, African-descent (black) nurses were needed in UK health care but were not 'wanted' in the UK. This discriminatory attitude underpins the current priority for international nurse recruitment from the Philippines and India (Donnelly, 2017) and, more recently, Nepal (Das, 2022). This preference for migrants with a lighter degree of skin pigmentation or 'shade' of skin is a determinant of discrimination (Allan and Larsen, 2003; Likupe, 2006), which builds on previous prejudice towards African descent migrant nurses.

Compared to the broader economy, the NHS has a higher proportion of staff from South Asia, Sub-Saharan Africa and South-East Asia (Barker, 2020) than the countries of China, India, Spain and the Philippines (Buchan et al., 2005), because UK health care employers can recruit nurses legally. As of January 2020, with 8,241 NHS staff members, Nigeria represents the most prominent African nation and the sixth-largest contributor to NHS staff behind the UK, India, Philippines, Ireland and Poland (Barker, 2020). A significant reason for not having recruitment agreements with countries in Sub-Saharan Africa, such as Nigeria, is the expressed concern about brain drain and depletion of human resources in the country's health care system. This excuse is shallow and does not tell the true story. There is a need to study how the international community may contribute to developing the workforce of the Sub-Saharan countries and continue to legally satisfy the requirement and recruitment of workforce from these countries into UK health care to resolve the problem of registered nurse shortage. In this 21st century, most of the raw materials for European industries are sourced from Africa without hesitancy. The material is used to service the industrial requirements in European nations, and the finished material is exported to Africa and sold at exorbitant prices. This practice has been the case since the days of colonialism and continues under neo-colonialism. Adeyeri and Adejuwon (2012: 1) argue that the

> colonial territory of Nigeria served not only as a ready source of cheap raw materials to feed the growing industries in Britain and European states but also as a trading post for the British and European traders and merchants and, at the same time, supported the importation of end-products because the British wanted an outlet for her own manufactured products to stave off declining domestic consumption and falling rate of profit at home.

My PhD (Ugiagbe, 2022) findings suggest that nurses trained in Nigeria pride themselves on speaking and writing English proficiently and do not have communication difficulties that they cannot resolve quickly. The historical link between the UK and Nigeria and respondents' confidence in having received formal education in the English language in Nigeria are significant factors in their choice of the UK as a destination country. My study suggests that Nigerian nurses' motivations to migrate to the UK support the equilibrium perspectives more than the 'push and pull' effect. It indicates that IEN migration is a planned and calculated measure to promote individual development and progress. The NMC imposition of discriminatory requirements for Anglophone African nurses in registration to practice in the UK is a deliberate challenge contributing to institutional discrimination and structural discrimination in the UK health care system for ethnic minority nurses. The registration body, since the establishment of the NHS, has streamlined the training and registration of IENs to practice in the UK to reflect the political policy on Immigration at any specific period and has therefore contributed mainly to the continuity of nurse shortage in the UK and the persisting issue of discrimination in UK health care. As argued above, IENs' English language competence or standard of nursing practice was not considered substandard from 1948 to the introduction of the language competence test in 2005., As Ugiagbe et al. (2022:1) argue, 'English language tests for ORNs seeking registration in the United Kingdom uare discriminatory due to the UK's racist migration policies and a regulatory body for nursing and midwifery that fails to acknowledge and understand its own institutionally racist practices'. In the light of this and other criticism of its racist practices (West et al., 2017), the NMC has now reviewed its requirement in 2023 for IENs to show satisfactory evidence through employers that the applicant's nurse training and assessment were in English to become NMC registered nurses (NMC, 2023). The success of this change depends on the willingness and commitment of employers and the NMC to implement robust plans without exorbitant cost to the IEN to affect the collation of the evidence required from IENs for the NMC.

Conclusion

In this chapter the history and challenges of the existing policies and procedures regarding IENs' recruitment, retention and integration has been discussed. I argue that the NMC has contributed to the continuity of nurse shortages in the UK and persisting discrimination in UK health care. In doing so, it has failed to criticise racist immigration policies. The health care system has been sustained by institutional racism. Alderwick and Allan (2019[1]) argue that the NHS needs more migrant staff and estimates that an additional 5,000 international nurses must be recruited yearly to sustain the NHS. There are other benefits derivable from transnational migration, such as improved sharing of health care knowledge, equipment and resources, development of exchange programmes and enhanced opportunity for improved bilateral and multilateral agreements on recruitment of international health professionals, respecting the freedom of health workers to migrate as well as circular or return migration for critical skills. The NMC is well placed to promote the benefit derivable from the international recruitment of nurses from erstwhile colonial countries of Africa.

Note

1 Since I wrote this chapter, we have seen the publication of the Conservative government's workforce plan for the NHS which recognises the deficit in the workforce.

References

Adeyeri, O., and Adejuwon, K. D. (2012, August). *International Journal of Advanced Research in Management and Social Sciences*, 1(2). www.garph.co.uk

Alderwick, H., and Allan, L. (2019). *Immigration and the NHS: The evidence*. https://www. health.org.uk/news-and-comment/blogs/immigration-and-the-nhs-the-evidence

Allan, H., and Larsen, J. A. (2003). *"We need respect": Experiences of internationally educated nurses in the UK*. London: RCN.

Allan, H. T., and Westwood, S. (2015). White British researchers and internationally educated research participants: Insights from reflective practices on issues of language and culture in nursing contexts. *Journal of Research in Nursing*, 20(8). https://doi.org/10.1177/1744987115618236

Allan, H. T., and Westwood, S. (2016). English language skills requirements for internationally educated nurses in the care industry: Barriers to UK registration or institutionalised discrimination? *International Journal of Nursing Studies*, 54, 1–4. https://doi.org/10.1016/j.ijnurstu.2014.12.006

Barker, C. (2020). *NHS staff from overseas: Statistics Number 7783*, 4th June, 2020. https://commonslibrary.parliament.uk/research-briefings/cbp-7783/

Batnitzky, A., and McDowell, L. (2011). Migration, nursing, institutional discrimination and emotional/affective labour: Ethnicity and labour stratification in the UK National Health Service. *Social and Cultural Geography*, 12(02), 181–201. doi: 10.1080/14649365.2011.545142

Berger, R. (2015). Now I see it, now I don't: Researcher's position and reflexivity in qualitative research. *Qualitative Research*, 15(2), 219–234. https://doi. org/10.1177/1468794112468475

Buchan, J., Jobanputra, R., Gough, P., and Hutt, R. (2005). *Internationally recruited nurses in London: Profile and implications for policy*. London: King's Fund.

Buchan, J. (2007). International recruitment of nurses: Policy and practice in the United Kingdom. *Health Services Research*, 42(3p2), 1321–1335.

Cousin, G. (2009). *Researching Learning in Higher Education*. Abingdon: Routledge.

Cummings, J. (2014). *Nurses are central to a transformation in care*. https://www. england.nhs.uk/blog/jane-cummings-5

Das, S. (2022). Overseas nurses in the UK forced to pay out thousands if they want to quit jobs. Nursing. *The Guardian*, 27th March, 2022.

Department of Health (DoH). (2000). *The NHS Plan: A Plan for Investment. A Plan for Reform*. HMSO.

Donnelly, L. (2017). *Number of EU nurses coming to UK falls 90 per cent since Brexit vote*. https://www.telegraph.co.uk/science/2017/01/25/number-eu-nurses-coming-uk-falls-90-per-cent-since-brexit-vote/9

Geddes, A. (2003). *The Politics of Migration and Immigration in Europe*. https:// www.researchgate.net/publication/288272904_The_Politics_of_Migration_and_ Immigration_in_Europe

Gentleman, A. (2022, May 29). The racist legislation that led to Windrush. *The Guardian*. https://www.theguardian.com/uk-news/2022/may/29/racist-legislation-led-Windrush-home-office

Henry, L. (2007). Institutionalized disadvantage: Older Ghanaian nurses' and midwives' reflections on career progression and stagnation in the NHS. *Journal of Clinical Nursing*, 16, 2196–2203.

Hilario, C., Browne, A. J., & McFadden, A. (2017). The influence of democratic racism in nursing inquiry. *Nursing Inquiry*, 25, e12213. https://doi.org/10.1111/nin.12213

Jayaweera, H. (2015). *Background Report: Migrant Workers in the UK Healthcare Sector*. Work-INT. COMPAS, School of Anthropology, University of Oxford.

Kirkham, R. S., and Anderson, J. M. (2002). Postcolonial nursing scholarship: From epistemology to method. *Advances in Nursing Science*, 25(1), 1–17.

Kofman, E. (1999). Female 'birds of passage' a decade later: Gender and immigration in the European Union. *International Migration Review*, 33(2), 269–299. https://doi.org/10.1177/019791839903300201

Likupe, G. (2006). Experiences of African nurses in the UK National Health Service: A literature review. *Journal of Clinical Nursing*, 15(10), 1213–1220.

Mann, S. (2016). *The Research Interview*. [Kindle Paper white]. Retrieved from http://www.amazon.co.uk/

McConnell-Henry, T., Chapman, Y, and Francis, K. (2009). Husserl and Heidegger: Exploring the disparity. *International Journal of Nursing Practice*, 15(1), 7–15.

Nexus Partnerships Limited. (2020). *The Commonwealth – Commonwealth of Nations: History of the Commonwealth*. History of the Commonwealth – Commonwealth of Nations

NHS Employers. (2017a). *NHS Workforce: Ethnicity Facts and Figures*. https://www.ethnicity-facts-figures.service.gov.uk/workforce-and-business/workforce-diversity/nhs-workforce/latest. Accessed 15/10/19.

NHS Employers. (2017b, December). *Language Competency: Good Practice for Employers*. http://www.nhsemployers.org/case-studies-and-resources/ 2017/12/language-competency-good-practice-guidance-for-employers

NMC (2019). *Changes announced to help boost nursing and midwifery workforce*. News Update. Date 21st March 2019. https://www.nmc.org.uk/news/news-and-updates/changes-announced-to-help-boost-nursing-and-midwifery-workforce/. Accessed 17/08/23

NMC (2023) Guidance on registration language requirements Updated June 2023. London. Nursing and Midwifery Council.

Nursing and Midwifery Council (NMC) (2015) *NMC Strategy 2015-2020*. Accessed 01/07/. https://www.nmc.org.uk/globalassets/sitedocuments/annual_reports_and_accounts/strategy-2015-2020.pdf

Nursing and Midwifery Council. (2017a). *English Language Requirements*. https://www.nmc.org.uk/registration/joining-the-register/English-language-requirements/

Nursing and Midwifery Council. (2017b). *NMC Registering as a Nurse or Midwife in the UK Information for Applicants Trained Outside the European Union or European Economic Area*. https://www. healthcareers.nhs.UK/explore-roles/nursing/information-overseasnurses

Nursing and Midwifery Council. (2018). *Future Nurse: Standards of Proficiency for Registered Nurses*. future-nurse-proficiencies.pdf (nmc.org.uk).

Nursing and Midwifery Council. (2020). *Information for Educators of Nursing Associates*. The Nursing and Midwifery Council (nmc.org.uk).

Peate, I., and Lane, J. (2017). A tale of two countries: Enrolled nurses in the UK and Gibraltar. British. *Journal of Healthcare Assistants*, 11(3). https://doi.org/10.12968/bjha.2017.11.3.140

Rafferty, A-M, Solano. D. (2007). The rise and demise of the colonial nursing service: British nurses in the colonies 1896-1966. *Nursing History Review*, 15(1): 147–154.

Reynolds, D. (2019). *Island Stories: Britain and Its History in the Age of Brexit.* Harper Collins Publishers.

Royal College of Nursing. (2003). *Here to Stay? International Nurses in the UK.* London: Royal College of Nursing.

Royal College of Nursing. (2017). *RCN Policy Position on Language Testing and Response to the NMC's New Guidance.* https://www.rcn.org.uk/professional-development/publications/pub-006508

Royal College of Nursing. (2019). Chronic Staff Shortages Could Compromise Aims of NHS Long. https://www.rcn.org.uk/news-and-events/news/chronic-staff-shortages-could-compromise-aims-of-nhs-long-term-plan-warns-rcn

Royal College of Nursing. (2020). *Staff Safety at Risk Unless Nursing Shortages Are Addressed.* https://www.rcn.org.uk/news-and-events/news/uk-staff-safety-at-risk-unless-nursing-shortages-are-addressed-170920

Shepherd, J. (2019). Timeline: The road to nurse registration in the UK. *Nursing Times.*

Smith, P. A., Allan, H., Henry, W. L., Larsen, J. A., and Mackintosh, M. A. (2006). *Valuing and Recognising the Talents of a Diverse Healthcare Workforce.* Report from the REOH Study: Researching Equal Opportunities for Overseas-trained Nurses and Other Healthcare Professionals. European Institute of Health and Medical Sciences, University of Surrey, the Open University and the Royal College of Nursing.

Snow, S., and Jones, E. (2011). Immigration and the national health service: Putting history to the forefront. *History and Policy*, 30.03.2011. https://www.research.manchester.ac.uk/portal/en/publications/immigration-and-the-national-health-service-putting-history-to-the-forefront(6302199a-b807-494e-8bc5-196aa79d2fd8)/export.html. Accessed 15/10/22.

Solano, D., and Rafferty, A. (2007). Can lessons be learned from history? The origins of the British imperial nurse labour market: A discussion paper. *International Journal of Nursing Studies*, 44(6), 1055–1063.

Spencer, I. (1997). *British Immigration Policy Since 1939: The Making of Multi-racial Britain.* London: Routledge.

Spencer, S. (2011). *The Migration Debate.* Policy Press/Bristol University Press.

Takeielts.britishcouncil.org. (2018). *Book Your Test.* https://takeielts.britishcouncil.org/locations/united-kingdom

Telegraph.co.uk. (2007). *Enoch Powell's Rivers of Blood Speech.* https://www.telegraph.co.uk/comment/3643823/Enoch-Powells-Rivers-of-Blood-speech.html

Thewlis, S. (2003). *Select Committee on Constitution Written Evidence: Memorandum by the Nursing and Midwifery Council.* https://publications.parliament.uk/pa/ld200304/ldselect/ldconst/68/68we53.htm

Ugiagbe, I. M. (2022). *Integration of Internationally Educated Nurses to the UK: The Lived Experience of Nurses with Nigerian Heritage in the London Region.* PhD thesis, Middlesex University.

Ugiagbe, I., Liu, L. Q., Markowski, M., and Allan, H. T. (2022, July 13). A critical race analysis of structural and institutional racism: Rethinking overseas registered nurses' recruitment to and working conditions in the United Kingdom. *Nursing Inquiry*. https://doi.org/10.1111/nin.12512

UKCC. (1999). *Report of the UKCC's Commission for Nursing and Midwifery Education.* Chair, Sir Leonard Peach; http://www.nmcorg.uk/nmc/main/publications/fitnessforpractice.pdf

Webb, B. (2000). Enrolled nurse conversion: A review of the literature. *Journal of Nursing Management*, 8, 115–120.

West, E., Nayar, S., Taskila, T., and Mustafa Al-Haboubi. (2017). *The Progress and Outcomes of Black and Minority Ethnic (BME) Nurses and Midwives through the Nursing and Midwifery Council's Fitness to Practise Process*. NMC Report.

Yu, X. (2008). Facilitating adaptation of international nurses: Need for an evidence-based transition and integration programme. *Home Health Care Management and Practice*, 20(2), 199–202.

7 An exploration of the experience of Black and Minority Ethnic nurse educators in UK universities

Donna Scholefield

Introduction

Institutional racism within higher education institutions (HEIs) is a recognised issue (Bhopal 2015; Equality and Human Rights Commission 2019; Universities UK 2020) and the experiences of black female academics are known to be poorer than their white female colleagues (Khan et al. 2019; Rollock 2019). The intersection of racism, sexism and class prejudice that black female academics can experience in higher education emerged as an important theme in the interview data that I present below. It influenced and reshaped my research question and the decision to analyse in more depth the following sections from the interview transcripts of one of the 12 participants from my PhD thesis entitled The *experience of black and ethnic minority nurse academics in higher education.*

This chapter was written through the lens of my own experience of racism in HEIs and how this research journey has helped me to articulate the racialised experience of black female academics. It will focus on one participant '*Pearl*' and on her experience of multiple sources of oppressions (racism, sexism, class based), a major theme that emerged. The findings will be informed by a dialogic/performance narrative methodology. The first section provides an overview of the methodology and my positionality within the research and the second an interrogation of the interview process, how the narrator's story emerges and my responses to it. Riessman (2008) suggests that the selection of segments of a narrative for detailed analysis should be guided by the research question(s) as this allows the researcher to 'infiltrate' the transcript by various means. To that end, data from Pearl's narrative will be presented in the form of excerpts and scenes structured using stanzas (Gee's 2011, 2014).

Methodology

A Dialogical/Performance (Riessman 2008) approach was used to interrogate Pearl's narrative data. This approach, Riessman contends, is broad and incorporates elements of both thematic and structural methods of analysis, which specifically *'interrogates'* discourses between the speakers (narrator

DOI: 10.4324/9781003269915-7

and interviewer) and is *'produced and performed as narrative.'* Important dimensions addressed in this method of analysis and that separate it from other types of qualitative analysis are: the close attention that is paid to the vocabulary, how segments of the data are organised, questioning why it is organised in this way; social positioning within the story (how the narrator positions herself, the audience, other characters within the story); the interactional context of the interview – accepting that the interviewer, audience, local, historical and social context, as well as other dimensions, all play an important part in shaping the narrative (Riessman 2016). Riessman's dialogic/performance approach also draws on **Goffman's Dramaturgical theory** (1981) which uses the metaphor of actors in a play to explain our everyday interactions with others. Goffman contends that like actors on a stage, we spend most of our lives performing on the 'front stage' delivering the most favourable side of ourselves to an audience, especially in difficult situations and it is only when 'back stage' i.e. at home or safe place that our true self is exposed.

Riessman (2008) argues that although Goffman's notion of performance is about enactment of the *'preferred self'* performance is also about a certain *'genre of talk'* when two speakers are in conversation with each other. There is a certain understanding and acceptance of the type of talk between the speakers not evident when they are some distance apart (Wolfson 1989). Gee (2014) suggests that an important question to ask in analysing research discourses is:

> ...*What knowledge, assumptions and inferences listeners have to bring to bear in order for this communication to be clear and understandable and received in the way the speaker intended?*
>
> (2014, pg 18)

Gee's (2011, 2014) approach was adapted to **structure and present the data** (Segment 1) concerning a significant event within Pearl's narrative by grouping the information firstly into larger sections (setting, catalyst, crisis, resolution and coda) what Gee refers to as the **macrostructure**. Then, within these sections, lines concerning a single topic are referred to as **stanzas** or microstructure of the story in particular. Gee contends that using this approach captures more elements of what a speaker is saying than the use of only a line of speech (Gee 2011, pg 137).

As a black female academic, I have also experienced multiple (racism, sexism, classism) forms of discrimination and could both empathise and sympathise with the experiences of many of the participants in my doctoral research. Although a few participants had a very positive journey, I found myself feeling saddened and angry at the end of interviews with those who had had adverse experiences. I could not remain unemotional and detached. My positioning as a peer and a BME academic has undoubtedly influenced my relationship with the participants and inevitably the telling of their stories. Some for example stated that they were more comfortable speaking with me about their experiences in HE and even asked questions at the end of the interview about my own experience of racism in the academy. Others like Pearl were eager for their stories to be told and wanted their experience to benefit a wider audience. Other BME scholars (Bhopal 2010) researching within this area have had similar experiences claiming, as I found, that it can enhance trust and empathy between participants and the researcher leading to a more open and honest dialogue. While interviews were conducted with as much impartiality as possible, Bamberg and Andrews (2004) concludes that this co-construction reflects the speakers' identities and what they think the audience (the interviewer) wants to hear or what they will find acceptable and worthwhile. Others (Charmaz 2006) however, would argue rather than a co-construction the stories are a reconstruction of reality. That said, the advantage of the methodology, according to Riessman (2008), is that it *'privileges positionality and subjectivity'* thus allowing me to infiltrate the narratives of these women and not feel guilty about objectivity as subjectivity is welcomed. I was, however, cognisant of my positionality throughout the stages of the research and the potential bias that this could impose on the analysis and interpretation of the data. See Box 7.1, Establishing Trustworthiness in narrative research.

Presentation one case: Academics experience within HEI

Pearl

Early years in Academia

Pearl is an experienced black female academic born in the UK of Jamaican descent. At the time of the interview, she was in her mid-50s working in her second HEI in the South of England.

We engaged in a long 2-hour interview which focused on stories of the racism she experienced. Pearl became a nurse after leaving school. She enjoyed her nursing course at a well-known teaching hospital forming lifelong friendships. Pearl made rapid progress within the clinical setting, securing several senior positions in the NHS. Her career direction changed as she became disillusioned as she felt her passion to effect change was being impeded by organisational structures and policies. So encouraged by the director of nursing, who Pearl stated was very supportive and thus a significant figure in her career, she became the in lead in Practice Development. This shifted her focus from management to education and staff development.

Pearl decided to move into education after completing her master's degree and teaching diploma. For the next ten years, Pearl enjoyed her role as senior lecturer in the nursing department, taking on a range of responsible positions, facing few challenges and felt supported in her endeavours within the department.

At this point in the interview, I remember scribbling in my notes that as a black person fully supported and comfortable in your bubble it can give a false sense of security about what other BME staff may be enduring.

Pearl described incidences of racial microaggression within the classroom while working as a lecturer (see extract below). These she infers were everyday occurrences which were dealt with swiftly and adeptly.

> ...it's [racism] always very subtle in a classroom and... 95% of the time, it's not an issue... But once you clearly identify where the power lies... or that... this is a collegiate room...we try to be respectful to everybody ...9.9 times out of 10, you drop some long words into a sentence that they [Students] don't understand that's related to nursing, you're pretty good really.

I felt that these incidents were not particularly significant to her, and Pearl's utterances in this excerpt indicate that they either had little emotional impact or that she did not want to acknowledge its effect. As others have suggested (Sue et al. 2007; Holder et al. 2015; Williams 2020) these everyday incidences have a cumulative effect and over time racial microaggressions inflict significant unconscious emotional damage and can lead to physical and mental health issues.

Pearl was also frustrated by the oppressive culture of the nursing department at that time, with its heavy focus on teaching and course management to the exclusion of other areas such as research.

> ...a conference... no senior member of staff ...at appraisal said anything to me about, or ..., any research ...you might be considering doing – those kinds of conversations didn't exist: 'is your module running well; are your students happy; is the fail rate low? – that's it.'... you've got 40 exams to mark and you think well, that will have to wait[Research], I haven't got time for that.

Despite feeling frustrated, Pearl enjoyed teaching, becoming more research aware through her involvement in a small research project and presenting the findings at a conference. However, a turning point in her awareness of discrimination within the department arose when she was invited to teach by the head of the sociology department in the summer school but was categorically refused by her manager.

> ('I won't support you', that's how she said it, 'I won't support you'; just like that')

This refusal angered Pearl because she felt that there was no sensible rationale for the decision.

Angry. [asked how she felt about refusal] Um, very angry and very shocked actually…

Racialised experience

When I asked if she felt this was a racialised incident, Pearl was equivocal. Her understanding, however, of these as racialised incidents emerged during the interview.

('I don't know if I want to pinpoint that down to racial discrimination…')

Another confrontation arose with her manager who refused to allow Pearl to complete her PhD, the reason given was that it was not sufficiently related to nursing.

'we <u>will not support you</u> in doing your PhD' (long pause) …[I] was like, 'really? – ok, ok!'… if you're saying to me, we're not going to support you because it's not a nursing related subject, for me, that's a 'black' thing, personally … 'Ok, this one, I was like, are you for real, really?! This time, I was thinking, you're taking the piss now; this time I was thinking, you know … I have the feeling that, if a male member of this staff came in and said to you, I want to look at the identify of white British men, she could have made that connection to nursing. That's why from this one, <u>**my gut is telling me it is a black thing**</u>, my gut is telling me that.

Pearl's reaction was one of intense anger and frustration, illustrated in the extract above by the use of expletives, expressions of surprise *(really, for real!)*, hand gestures and repetition of emotive phrases, at the unfairness and irrationality of the decision. Given the focus of the PhD, Pearl was convinced that the grounds for this refusal was racial discrimination *(my gut is telling me it is a black thing…')*.

Pearl concluded that her manager was discriminatory. Indeed, one particular utterance that resonated with me during Pearl's description of her interaction with manager was the following *'That's why from this one, my gut is telling me it is a black thing, my gut is telling me that.'* Here I believe she was struggling to fully rationalise the behaviour of her manager but it seems her intuition, based on a lifetime of experiencing discrimination, was telling her it was racism.

This last encounter changed Pearl's perception of the organisation, heightening awareness of structural racism in this particular university.

Yes, '… <u>it was a significant</u>, that was the <u>beginning of the end for me at this university</u>, … the 10 years that I'd worked here with not much problems, doing my job more than competently at least ... didn't mean anything at all... **Excerpt 5**.

She left the university, angry and embittered at being belittled and disrespected

... obviously, those qualifications that got me my position [MSc, BSc, professional qualifications], you're negating those then; my academic qualifications ... what I do have an issue with is respect...being used and inconsistency;

In summary, this section reviewed Pearl's early years in academia. She enjoyed her early years but became frustrated with thwarted career progression, the oppressive nature of her department, and the racialised encounters with one of her white managers. She left this university angry and embittered because she felt exploited and disrespected. The following section (Segment 1) will analyse multiple intersecting discriminations that Pearl encounters in her second HEI.

Segment 1: Pearl – Analysis-fighting against overt and covert discrimination

At the time of the interview, Pearl had been working at her second and current HEI for three years she describes what happened when she was interviewed, whilst in her probationary year, as a preliminary measure to commence her PhD studies by a panel headed by the Dean of her school. The research question had now been reformulated so that it was directly related to nursing and she was assured by the panel when interviewed for her present post that she could begin this programme of study if she was offered the post. In addition, she had the full support of her line manager to begin her studies as soon as possible.

As displayed in these scenes (Segment 1) the meeting resulted in an ill-tempered exchange between Pearl and the Dean because he felt the topic and the research question was an inappropriate choice and was adamant that she could not commence it in her probationary year. This is despite a verbal agreement at her interview and support from her managers to commence her PhD studies. In the resolution scene of the story Pearl, against the Dean's wishes, commenced her PhD.

The transcript is divided into scenes. Pearl has created a number of characters – the Dean, her head of department, his managers, and given them all speaking roles including herself. Nonetheless, although there are other players it is very clear that Pearl positions herself at the very centre of the whole narrative, once again accentuating her sense of agency and control within her story. Throughout this segment, linguistic devices such as expressive language, direct speech are employed to dramatise the performance. In these scenes Pearl seeks to make sense of yet another rejection. She is convinced that racism and sexism are the reasons for rejection by the Dean.

*Segment 1: Pearl – Analysis-Fighting against overt
and covert discrimination*

Scene 1. Perception racial discrimination

1 '…yeah, so my current university I can say, for a first time in a long, long, long, long, long time, where **it's** been, 100% [Referring to Racism]
2 I have no problem in saying **it**, was completely **and totally racially motivated,**
3 it was all forms of racism:
4 so it was **institutional racism;** … racial discrimination; there was a whole **gender issue**

Scene 2

1 well – let's get into **intersectionality** –
2 Yeah, yeah, *you know, you know,* class,
3 you know, overt, covert racism, I mean, **wooo!**;
4 it was every single type of microaggression, every type of **racism** that you could possibly imagine, I experienced in that place.

Scene 3

1 So institutional racism would be, um, you apply for your PhD,
2 …your manager and your manager's manager are fully aware of, and 100% behind you… and those are two white people, cannot fault them… you apply, as directed by them,

Scene 4. Catalyst

1 and you go and you sit in front of a panel
2 and the Head of the panel is the Dean of the **School!**, sorry, yeah, the Dean of the **School!**
3 And he says to you, *'this topic area is not a PhD,'* that's what he says.
4 …Now, again [Dean repeats assertion] – and *you're on probation at this point, you know, just started here …so you can't do a PhD on your probation.*
5 This man does **not have a PhD**
6 this man is a radiographer by history.

Scene 5. Unsupportive women.

1 And every other white woman, sat at that desk, does not disagree with him,
2 and two of **those women** have a PhD,

Scene 6. Perception of institutional racism

1 So we have **overt racism**, because he's telling a black woman that a PhD, that now has nursing in it, so it's nursing related now, and it's about British born Caribbean women;
2 it's about **black nurses and their nursing identity**,
3 and he says it's not a PhD.
4 So, I'm sorry, if a **white, middle-class man** says that to me, that's racist.
5 **Institutionally**, you can't do it in the first year, when you're on probation.
6 Where is that written? Nowhere.
7 it clearly tells them in your personal, in your statement, … at interview, what you want to do, and what it's gonna be on,
8 So it's not written anywhere, that you can't do that[PhD]…'
9 That's institutional racism;
10 you are **using the systems and processes of your organisation to**
11 **block a black person from doing what they should be doing,**

Scene 7. Bullying tactics

1 it's overtly be **aggressive towards me**, based on the fact **that I'm a black woman** and I will not back down… there are nurses of various ethnic groups in our dept that are doing nursing, that work in this dept. *Why is my PhD not a PhD? Again*
2 So every trick in the book to *demean, degrade and disrespect* me, is brought out.

Scene 8. Feelings

1 This [Asked how this made her feel], well I was –
2 I think I actually said it to my manager – **incandescent with rage, is the word I used,**
3 **because it was just so overt,**
4 and I told my **white male manager that. It** took him a while,

Scene 9. Other characters perception

1 it's taken two attempts at me finally getting my funding and everything,
2 that he [manager] doesn't try to question that statement anymore[Overt racism].
3 Because he did try to defend it: he doesn't say, I agree with you Pearl; what he does now is that he doesn't say anything, and so in my world, in my mind, that means he agrees with me now.

Scene 10. White liberals

1 Um, he tried to defend it –
2 again, in the way that **white liberals try to defend it.**
3 So he moved it away from that
4 and said about, you know, I don't necessarily think it was that[Racism],

5 and then **I gave him the reasons I've just given you,**
6 ...and he said *'I don't see colour,'*
7 **God love him, bless him!**
8 **And a white liberal thinks that's a good thing to say when –**
9 **it's like saying I have a black friend,**
10 **it's not necessarily a good thing to say!**
11 Um, you know, and **I don't see any difference,**
12 and I said to him, well, actually, there is a difference:
13 you're a *white man and I'm a black woman;* that's a difference.
14 And that's *not a problem;*
15 *it's the power of distribution within that, that's the problem.*

Scene 11

1 Do you know what I mean?
2 So I've got, so the Dean of the School is a white man
3 and he said a PhD that's got nursing in the title is not a PhD – **he doesn't have a PhD.**
4 What am I supposed – as a black woman, there's no other thing that I'm going to think –

Scene 12. Credibility

1 I said, I'm an experienced lecturer, I said I was a senior nurse before I came into nursing,
2 I said I've had my degree and my masters from... University ... of London.
3 ... you hide me because of my experience, and then I **stand in a room full of my peers** and the man looks at me and says it's not a PhD.

Scene 13. Stalemate

1 Well, I made it very clear to him that I wasn't happy,
2 and he made it very clear that he wasn't happy ...
3 and I don't really give a damn,
4 and about half-way through the meeting, I stopped talking.

Scene 14. Resolution

1 and I already had in my mind, I will apply for my PhD..., like I planned.
2 And that's exactly what I did.

Analysis

Pearl's perception of racialised and sexist behaviour

In scenes 1–3 Pearl forcefully and dramatically expresses the many types of racism that she feels she has encountered in her interaction with the Dean – including racial microaggressions and institutional racism. Clearly, as revealed in scene 4, the catalyst for her anger was being blocked from commencing her PhD by a man without a doctorate and who was unable to provide a cogent argument for his decision. The narrative infers he lacked both the credibility and the authority to make such a decision.

Pearl's reading of this situation (and mine) is that this was a white man in a position of power who would dominate the exchange and she would be the one that would have to succumb to his hegemony. Paradoxically she is the one in the narrative that is in control of the situation *('...I will not back down...)* and instead of succumbing she fights back (S: 7–13) and reiterates the arguments for why she is entitled to do her PhD. Casting the Dean as a weak and vulnerable character, having no sound arguments to support his position except to repeat the same phrases – *'this topic area is not a PhD, ... and you're on probation.'* In the resolution scene (14) Pearl demonstrates her contempt and lack of respect for the Dean by ignoring him and beginning her programme of study.

Pearl's emphatic response is bolstered by other characters, such as the head of the department and his immediate manager whom she positions as being both sympathetic and supportive of her. In addition, her sociological (MSc) background, specifically her knowledge and understanding of racism and critical race theory (CRT), enabled her cogent processing and evaluation of the discourse dynamics. This is evident in the vocabulary used throughout this segment.

There are, however, consequences for victims of microaggression in fighting back. Her reaction enraged the Dean further as his authority became increasingly under threat (scene 7). Pearl infers that the Dean became aggressive and perpetuated racially microaggressive behaviour. In another meeting that resulted in another angry exchange with the Dean, Pearl describes the Dean directing racial micro assaults towards her.

> ...And then, he started personally attacking me in the way I was communicating and gesticulating...

So although there is little detail about the exchange in scene 7 there is sufficient information in the whole of this segment 1 and other segments of the narrative for the audience to infer a negative outcome. This manifests as an escalation in the argument and racial micro assaults (Sue et al. 2007). By attacking Pearl's hand gestures and speech, these actions (according to Sue et al. (2007)) are the Dean's attempt, to *'pathologise'* Pearl's *cultural values*. Signifying that he felt Pearl's communication method was abnormal is a personal attack and the Dean is unwittingly disclosing his stereotypical views about a person of colour. This type of racial microaggression is classified as a racial microassault (Sue 2010; Sue et al. 2007) and is usually a conscious, explicit and deliberate attempt to hurt the intended victim. Certainly, he succeeded as the injury inflicted by the hurt and anger is conveyed in Pearl's utterances and how she frames segment 1.

Intersectionality and Bullying behaviour in the higher education sector

Bullying is also evident in this segment (Scene: 7, 10) and others in the narrative *(attacking how she was communicating)* that Pearl casts the Dean as being unpleasant – *aggressively dominant and coercive*, all from a position of *power* (Keashly & Neuman, 2010). An imbalance of social power was evident, here as he knew he had the authority to prevent Pearl from commencing her PhD.

Given Pearl's descriptions of racial microaggressions and bullying in her interactions with the Dean, I felt that it could be argued that gender discrimination was also evident. I was reminded of Bhopal's (2019) contention that the intersectionality of social identities such as sex, and ethnicity is central to the positionality of black females in academia. His actions could therefore be perceived as attempts to hinder her progress and uphold the status quo through marginalisation and male patriarchy (Jensen 2021).

Racial trauma

Pearl suggests in the narrative that the Dean's behaviour may have been motivated by resentment and insecurity, such as being the head of the department and not having a PhD. Pearl casts the Dean in several scenes [Segment 1] as a one-dimensional archetypal villain in the plot.

Audiences may well empathise as I did with this portrayal because the narrative suggests there is an intention by the Dean to cause harm which according to Neuman and Baron (2005) is a defining characteristic of bullying. Certainly, this part of the narrative clearly reveals/discloses Pearl's hurt and anger. This puts the Dean in a position of strength and Pearl in one of weakness. Here she is the victim because in these scenes he is the initiator of the anger and frustration she is feeling. Pearl articulates throughout the narrative the anger she was feeling but I sensed by her behaviour in the telling that the most poignant moments for Pearl were the personal attacks by the Dean. Such as when he attempted to belittle her by attacking her verbal and non-verbal communication style.

The fact that she expresses her anger throughout the narrative so viscerally, even though these incidents had taken place many years before the interview, is suggestive of what Williams (2020) refers to as *racial-based trauma*, the traumatic stress experienced by black and ethnic minority individuals as a result of sustained exposure to racism and discrimination.

> ...I have not moved away from the anger, I'm gonna be honest; I'm going to be angry about that for a very, very long time. ...

Feeling of isolation in a predominantly white space

In scene 5 I felt there was some evidence of Pearl's vulnerability. For example, when the whole panel remained silent including the females present on the panel whilst the dean persisted with his irrational behaviour.

> ...every other white woman, sat at that desk, does not disagree with him, and two of those women have a PhD, ... [T4 Scene 5. Lines 26–29].

Pearl at that moment must have felt very lonely and isolated and her comments at that moment would undoubtedly illicit the empathy of the audience.

Summary

This section has provided some insight into Pearl's experience of the intersection of racism (both overt and subtle) and sexism and how she chooses to interpret and respond to these oppressions. I feel her response in this segment was perceptive, articulate and robust. For example her astuteness in noting the reaction of the white female panellists inferring their collusion in her isolation (Bhopal et al. 2016; Rollock 2019). These observations also reveal Pearl's knowledge and insight into race and feminist scholarly literature. This deduction is reinforced by utterances within other segments of her narrative. Indeed, in the latter part of the interview when I asked about support systems for new lecturers; Pearl's words are clear about where the balance of power in HEI lies.

> **Reflection**
>
> It's interesting but in this scene (5) where she comments on the reaction of the women on the panel, I felt that Pearl's positioning changes from her predominant situated identity of a strong agentic black woman to a more passive vulnerable one. It demonstrates fluidity in her performance thus supporting Riessman's (2008) contention that the roles narrators allocate to themselves in not fixed. These fluctuations according to Harre and van Langenhove (1999) help the narrator '...*to cope with the situations they find themselves in*'

> ...find a white person, cause...it's like 99% chance that that person that's gonna support you is going to be a white person... it doesn't matter how high up... even as a black person...you are going to have to come up with a senior person who is white and they will take another senior person who is white, more seriously.

Dramatisation of Pearl's performance

As discussed earlier in this chapter, there are linguistic and behavioural performative features that can be identified in Pearl's narratives that serve to dramatise a particular performance (Cussins 1998). Pearl's utterances about racist incidents are linguistic features (direct speech, metaphors, expressive sounds, repetitions asides) that dramatise the events and serve to draw the audience into the story. Furthermore, she employs the use of direct speech to her characters and herself when highlighting important aspects of the narratives.

Examples direct speech:
Dean
    "this topic area is not a PhD... and you're on probation at this point, you know, just started here ...so you can't do a PhD on your probation. *(Scene 4)*
Managers:
    he said, " ... I don't see colour...' (Scene 10)
Pearl
    "Why is my PhD not a PhD again?" (Scene 7).

Pearl's use of direct reported speech (Riessman 2008) makes the listener more inclined to believe her utterances as it adds 'credibility' to her utterances about the behaviour of the dean and other characters. For example, the use of direct reported speech phrase "I don't see colour" by her manager reinforces her position in the interaction and allows the white people present to *'feel good and have a clear conscience'* about the everyday racial injustices that black people suffer (Delgado & Stefancic 2017) The directness of the phrase legitimises racism by adding credibility to the assertions that her white male manager is a 'white liberal' and a racist (These terms have been explained in Chapter 1). The use of a powerful metaphor such as *'racism, has hit me like a train'* in a later exchange with the Dean, serves also to not only persuade but ensure the audience feels the full force of what Pearl is experiencing.

There are other linguistic features used by Pearl which dramatise and further engage the listener. The use of repetition (Riessman 2008) highlights important points in the narrative. Phrases are repeated numerous times throughout segment 1: *'not a PhD' 'you cannot do a PhD' 'it' a not a PhD'*

Pearl also uses asides, where she moves away from the thread of the narrative to speak directly to the audience (me). Below, Pearl is in her manager's office, angry, pacing around the room, shocked at the overt racism demonstrated by the dean. She then digresses and speaks directly to the audience [black people] as they will empathise

... all of, you know, in the background, you know, the normal things, the microaggressions...

The expressive sounds that Pearl makes within her utterances also serve to dramatise ('*...I mean wooo!' Scene 2*) her narrative (Riessman 2008) and flags up focal points in the narrative – '*...well – let's get into intersectionality – Yeah, yeah, you know, you know, class, you know, overt, covert racism, I mean, wooo!*' Here Pearl is signalling how shocked she is at the overt demonstration (as she perceives it) of racism, sexism and classism.

Another device Pearl uses is to switch tense (Wolfson 1989) stories are normally communicated in the past tense. Pearl uses verb tenses performatively by alternating the past with the present. What Wolfson refers to as the '*conversational historic present pg 138*'

> 'So I am now doing a PhD that merges my nursing and my sociology side.
>
>   I informed you on my application and at the interview, that I wanted to start my PhD within the year'
>
> 'Um, you know, and I don't see any difference ...and I said to him, well, actually, there is a difference: 'you're a white man and I'm a black woman; that's a difference (scene 10)
>
> ' 'I had filled in the paperwork that I'm supposed to, and I submitted something. The PhD topic area has nursing in it – I am a nurse –

These exchanges serve to enliven Pearl's performances and draw the audience into her narrative. There is another purpose which is to accentuate Pearl's agency (Riessman 2008). Indeed 'enactment' Goffman (1974, pg 5) states '*... is something that listeners can empathetically insert themselves into, vicariously re-experiencing what took place.*' Through these devices, the experience becomes poignant and emotional for both the narrator and the speaker. The engagement serves to generate a '*two-way narrative contract between teller and audience.*' (Langellier 2001, pg 150).

In summary, this section has analysed some of the features that are present in performed stories that serve to dramatise the performance.

How Pearl positions me

Pearl positions me as an '*insider,*' casting me in a range of roles, which to some extent influences how she performs in the scenes. For example, there are occasions where she positions me as a fellow Jamaican and segues into Jamaican patois using the word '*stupidness*' meaning it is nonsense. '*I can't think of any other reason apart from racism for that stupidness.*'

Other times I am positioned as a fellow nursing academic with insider knowledge of both the NHS and higher educational processes. Pearl made assumptions about the knowledge and insights I had as a listener. There is an assumption that I understand the jargon used within these institutions in order for us to communicate clearly and effectively. Pearl uses a number of terms that also assumes I have an understanding of race and ethnicity scholarly literature.

Pearl's situated identity in these scenes is that of a knowledgeable scholar of race literature and as such one that should be respected. So throughout the narrative references are made to terms such *as 'intersectionality' 'institutional racism' 'racial micro aggression' 'white liberal'* In the scene (Segment 1 scene 10) where Pearl discusses the thinking of white liberals, in order to understand the significance to Pearl of the following interaction between herself and the dean the *audience* would require some knowledge of CRT (Delgado & Stefancic 2017), *colour-blind racism* (Bonilla-Silva 2014) and the phenomenon of white fragility (Diangelo 2018) to have an understanding of why Pearl is offended by comments such *as ' I don't see colour' 'I have a black friend'*

Colour-blindness

Scene 10 depicts Pearl's manager's attempts to justify the behaviour of the Dean. He is initially sceptical about Pearl's accusation of individual and institutional racism but as her utterances infers, he eventually ceases to defend the Dean and in doing so distances himself from the behaviour of the Dean. Unfortunately, he does so by making a cliched defensive response (*'I don't see colour'*) which Pearl interprets as a racial microaggressive comment. Pearl's utterances, however, imply sympathy for her manager (*'... God love, bless him'*) proceeding to educate him (Scene 10 Line...) about the inappropriateness of his response and why it is important to acknowledge differences.

In this scene, Pearl's positioning of the manager is that of a victim putting him on the defensive. She may well be sympathetic towards him as I sense that she feels her manager's intentions were honourable in attempting to persuade Pearl that he was not racist and that he embraced key values of the university such as diversity. However, *'colour-blindness'* or colour-blind ideology some CRT scholars would argue 'legitimises racism' in that it ignores the suffering that people of colour experience on a daily basis, and at the same time upholds white hegemony. Pearl's manager's defensive response also supports Diangelo (2018) arguments that many white people exhibit defensive responses, verbal and non-verbal, in order to deal with *'racial stress'* coining this term as white fragility. Others would argue that it is important to acknowledge differences because not to do so is patronising and insulting, because it ignores the suffering of black people and denies the fact that white people are in a privileged position in this society. In short colour-blind ideology is the antithesis of structural racism. Pearl's linguistic pattern in this scene may also reflects Diangelo's contention that white people, even *'white liberals'* (Pearl's description of her manager) often express incredulity when black people talk about different forms of racism.

It should be acknowledged that in truth everyone sees differences based on the fact that most people have some sort of preconceived idea about different ethnic groups. In short, the form of telling in this scene is an example of how Pearl could be confident that her performance would be received by an audience [me and the wider academy] as she intended.

Discussion

Pearl's utterances concerning her first ten years of working within HEI portrayed contentment. Focussing on her teaching and managerial role, she progressed to programme lead with support from managers and a strong network of friends. But her narrative portrayed a department with a strong focus on teaching and cursory interest in staff development or research. Consequently, Pearl became disillusioned with the culture within the department. Interestingly, other participants in the study voiced similar concerns in their narrative maintaining that such a culture stifled intellectual ambition. Then when she sought to widen her interest and the department's reaction was to, in her view, thwart her development Pearl became discontented and her awareness of discriminatory practices within HE heightened. So, the catalyst appears to be discriminatory treatment by individuals in positions of power (In the first and second HEI) that led to an awareness of the significance of intersecting identities on the positioning of black female academics in HEI (Bhopal & Preston 2012).

Although early in the narrative there was some equivocation and reluctance to attribute unfair treatment to racially motivated behaviour, a response noted in studies in the literature (Bhopal et al. 2016), Pearl's understanding of these as racialised incidents emerged during the interview. Her narrative became unequivocal. It explicitly portrays a belief that the culture within HEIs remains a white hegemonic patriarchy with black female academics, regardless of their seniority, still facing racism, sexism and bullying (Rollock 2019). Furthermore, Pearl's utterances undoubtedly convey her conviction about whiteness as an ideology, who is valued and where the power lies in academia.

> '...find a white person, cause...it's like 99% chance that that person that's gonna support you is going to be a white person... it doesn't matter how high up... even as a black person...you are going to have to come up with a senior person who is white and they will take another senior person who is white, more seriously.'

Curiously, in the early part of her career, Pearl does not focus on how to circumvent the discrimination she later awakens but this development may well reflect Bhopal and Preston (2012) conception of the 'dynamic' nature of intersectionality and the notion that our identities is:

> ...a journey, one that changes through different times in history and transforms in different spaces.'
>
> (Bhopal & Preston 2012, pg 1)

Intersectionality, bullying and power balance in higher education

In the analysis section, Pearl portrayed the white Dean as an unpleasant bullying character (aggressive and coercive) abusing his power. This, however, is not surprising given that supervisors and senior administrators (people in positions of power) are often identified as bullies in academia (Keashly & Neuman 2010) and bullying within the HE sector (Keashly & Neuman 2010), like racism, is a common and underreported issue (Equality and Human Rights Commission 2019; Universities UK 2020). This is also applicable to the bullying of black female academics (Bhopal 2015; Rollock 2019). Kearshly and Neuman's detailed review of the literature cites higher prevalence of bullying in the UK HE sector (10%–20%) compared with other parts of the western world such as Scandinavian countries (2%–5%) and the United States (10%–14%).

Bhopal's (2014) findings exploring the experience of black and ethnic minority academics in senior positions in both the UK and US support the unequal power dynamics revealed in Pearl's narrative. Namely, that power within academia resides with a small group of middle-class, predominantly male, white academics. That said there was no support from the women sitting on the panel with the Dean. '*And every other white woman, sat at that desk, does not disagree with him, and two of those women have a PhD, ...*' and it is interesting that Pearl noted this response from her white colleagues and was not hesitant about vocalising it. Pearl's utterances in this excerpt I felt eloquently capture her feelings of alienation/isolation. Unfortunately, the findings of this thesis are not unique and are corroborated by other studies (Bhopal et al. 2016; Rollock 2019). I would also argue that the deference shown by the white women on that panel is yet another means by which some white female academics marginalise black academics. But I believe the incident also illustrates the oppressive intersection of gender and race. There is clearly a power differential as illustrated by the somewhat submissive behaviour of the women on the panel towards the Dean who by virtue of his gender and race holds the power in the hierarchy of academia. Rollock (2019) also argues in her qualitative study of the experience of twenty black female professors that white women deliberately othering their black female colleagues by '*kowtowing*' to men shines a negative light on white feminism because their behaviour is '*reinforcing a gendered and racialised hierarchy*' which she believes privileges white men and puts their black female colleagues in a disadvantageous position. In contrast, curiously other studies (Williams & Sharif 2021) exploring Allyship found that people with marginalised identities (e.g. females) were more likely to be true racial allies, because of their experience of oppression creating greater empathy with people of colour. Specifically, the researchers found that female participants had a significantly higher Allyship score than male (white) participants.

Situated identity

The proposed **socially situated identity of Pearl,** informed by Goffman's dramaturgical model, is essentially that of a strong confident determined black woman who will not let institutional racism break her. Pearl has agency and is not a passive character placing herself at the centre of the performance. Her narrative clearly communicates this is the predominant way that Pearl positions herself to herself and the audience. There is of course some fluidity in her positioning, as discussed earlier, and there are scenes where vulnerability is exposed (scene 4–7). Though Pearl uses a number of strategies to make sense of and process rejections by prominent individuals within the academy either through the lens of theoretical frameworks such as CRT, her own experience of racism, as well as through her academic writings and publications. So, one of the messages of the narrative is to raise awareness of the intersecting oppressions experienced by BME female academics within HE and how armed with the appropriate knowledge and support these women can surmount discrimination and prevail.

What did Pearl want to accomplish from her narrative?

The preceding sections focussed on evidence of the dramatisation of much of Pearl's narrative, particularly those parts of her discourse relating to experiences of structural intersectionality. This then raises the question of why Pearl chose to frame these sections of her story in this way. She could have just reported her narrative in a factual way as she did in earlier sections of the narrative where her utterances seemed less dramatic, and understated and more about the reporting of events, for example, circumstances that led to her becoming a nurse and her career trajectory within the clinical setting. This largely understated factual retelling is in contrast with other sections discussed above which are highly dramatised where she presents a performed story.

Narrative scholars agree that narratives are not just a record of past events but are framed, consciously or unconsciously (Freeman 2002), in the way they are specifically for the listener or invisible audiences to *accomplish* something. In other words, to have an effect (Riessman 2016 in Silverman pg 368). For Pearl, this performance had to be framed in a dramatic – even evangelical – performance. She needed to be an enthusiastic evangelist to get her message across, not just to me, but to a wider invisible audience of other black academics or perhaps all *black women* out there who suffer discrimination. Gee (2014) suggests that in the analysis of any communication the speaker may be trying to do more than one thing. I believe Pearl is trying to accomplish the following:

i   to increase awareness amongst a wider audience (academia and the public) that overt racism still exists within academia especially towards black women academics because the power within institutions is still dominated by a white male elite, so it is not just about addressing racism but the intersection of factors such gender, and class;

ii that policies in place within the academia such as Athena Swan benefits only white women not black women (Bhopal 2015)

iii to show other black women that through self-awareness and knowledge they can address the intersection of race, gender and class (Hill & Bilge 2016) and that this can be successfully confronted in HEI.

I feel Pearl wants a clear political message delivered – not just to me but to a much wider audience. Maybe Pearl's motive as Goffman argues was to achieve a personal goal of standing up to white hegemony and thus to maintain a consistent and positive preferred identity of a confident, black woman capable of resolutely and successfully confronting discrimination.

Experience of academia – Impact on Pearl – Reshaping her life – reimaging of her identity

I sense that on a personal level the retelling of these events perhaps acted as some sort of release from some of the emotions that she was experiencing. Arthur Frank noted that *'stories repair the damage that illness has done to people's sense of where they are in their lives. Stories are a way of redrawing maps and finding new destinations (Frank 1995, pg 54–55).* Although the quote is in reference to illness (Frank had a myocardial infarction and cancer) the narrative suggests that these events had a profound effect on Pearl's emotional state. Studies (Paradies et al. 2015; Bhui et al. 2018; Williams 2020) have clearly demonstrated the detrimental physical and mental health effects caused by sustained racism (racial trauma). When perpetrators of racism blame or deny marginalised groups of having racialised experiences, it intensifies the trauma (Polanco-Roman et al. 2016).

Certainly, Pearl's experiences have been instrumental in reshaping aspects of her life; however, I do not believe narrating these events fully repaired the damage caused by these racialised experiences. When asked how she now felt about these events which occurred some years ago, Pearl stated defiantly and demonstrably that she was *'still angry'* despite the fact that the events facilitated successful and rewarding outcomes. Certainly, how Pearl chose to frame the narrative – a dramatic and enraged enactment – of these racialised encounters supports this interpretation. Nevertheless, as a strong, confident, knowledgeable black woman – the preferred identity that Pearl positions herself with – one can succeed against a powerful and privileged male white elite. So, in a sense, the message from the narrative is a sort of a *'David and Goliath'* moral lesson.

Pearl's enactment of events in her narrative is dramatic, angry, emotive and unreserved and what I believe these segments from her narrative have provided is some insight into her personal experiences in academia and the

impact of oppressive intersecting identities as well as the oppressive and restrictive culture of the nursing departments.

Certainly, Pearl's narrative infers that these traumatic experiences have re-
composed her life and produced a reimagining of her identity as an academic.
So, these traumatic events appear to have focussed her interest on the plight
of black female academics, expanding her sphere of thinking and resulting
in a fierce desire to understand and expose discrimination. Furthermore, although other events (i.e. a partner with an academic background-doctorate;
teaching experience in other departments in the university), in her life, ignited
her interest in the world of research the narrative infers that she channelled
the anger that emerged from racialised experiences by immersing herself in
the world of research. A world she is clearly delighted to be a part of and
contribute to. Her utterances also infer that these traumatic experiences were
an awakening and are cast as an **epiphany** – a revelation. Pearl is clearly en-
joying her new positioning within academia.

> '...And that was the start for me with regards to doing more research...
>
> I enjoyed the whole research process – collecting the data and all that
> boring stuff, I **enjoyed that** –
>
> I've been to lots and lots of conferences since then...and I started
> doing other research on other things: more educational research that I
> did...And once you start going to conferences, you get more confident
> about going to conferences...'

Her narrative infers that the strong emotional responses, specifically the anger she felt, resulting from racialised experiences, provided the impetus for
her interest and immersion into the world of research.

Trustworthiness

My position as a black female academic (See introduction) will invariably
influence my analysis and interpretation of the findings but as discussed previously the dialogic/performance approach according to Riessman (2008)
'privileges positionality and subjectivity.' Nevertheless, the importance of
trustworthiness in research is essential and Riessman (1993) asserts that there
are strategies that researchers can employ to demonstrate this (see Box 7.1).

The case study (Box 7.1) illustrates that other voices should be considered
in a narrative text. Indeed, Bakhtin (Dentith 1995) reminds us narrative texts
are polyphonic (multi-voiced). He contends that in a dialogic environment,
there are many voices besides that of the narrator each voice with its own
perspectives, equal weighting and validity. Therefore, the voice of the narrator should not be taken as the final authority on the text. So, when analysing
a personal narrative, it is the role of the analyst to examine not only the voice
of the narrator, but utterances of characters in the plot for 'hidden discourses'
gaps, ambiguities, disparities and divergences. That said Pearl firmly believed

---

Box 7.1   Establishing trustworthiness in narrative

Case study 1 Director of nursing refusal to support Pearl's PhD application

Riessman (1993) contends that one approach that the narrative scholar can use to establish the trustworthiness of the narrative is by finding the evidence from the transcripts that support the arguments as well as endeavouring to put forward alternatives that may promote trustworthiness. However, Czarniawska (2010, pg 402) argues it is not just a matter of 'quoting literally' but what is important is resituating sections of narrative that are trustworthy and thought-provoking *'it is a question of recontextualisation that is interesting, credible and respectful.'*

So, is there any conceivable evidence in Pearl's statements or the way she frames her narrative that could suggest an alternative hypothesis besides racial discrimination? Gee (2014) maintains that sometimes what people unconsciously say may betray their thoughts, so could another explanation for the director of nursing's refusal to support Pearl commencing her PhD be an unconscious display of vindictiveness because her authority has been undermined previously by a more senior colleague in overruling her decision not to allow Pearl to teach in another department? She could offer no concrete rationale for refusing to allow Pearl to commence a doctorate except that nursing did not appear in the title of her thesis. Pearl, when asked about the possibility of previous disputes with the director of nursing, did admit that there was an issue in the past her response indicated that this was some time ago and she now had a respectful professional relationship but from the response, I would suggest a detached and distant relationship.

> '...there was an issue, back in the day, but, even then, ... I just don't engage with that person [Director of Nursing] ... and when I did, I was professional...'

So, the decision by her manager to block Pearl could simply be an act of revenge for a perceived past slight. If this was the underlying reason, then her behaviour demonstrates a lack of professionalism and an abuse of power.

---

she was being victimised. This according to CRT scholars (Delgado & Stefancic 1993) is her *'reality.'* Furthermore, others (Sue et al. 2019; Williams 2020) contend that it is the individuals who are exposed to racism and racial microaggression that are best placed to accurately assess racist acts rather than the observer or the privileged perpetrators of these acts.

Despite challenges such as structural racism and the inequity in the power relationships in academia that female academics face on a daily basis, black female academics are resilient and have devised many survival strategies. Pearl is very much aware of the perception that **women** particularly black women are still seen as *'belonging outside power.'* This perception according to Mary Beard (2018 pg 56) is very apparent today and is underscored by the many metaphors that we as a society use when declaring women's access to power. Nonetheless, until black female academics like Pearl develop critical consciousness, then the inequity in the power relationships within academia will persist

Finally, my sense from reading and interrogating Pearl's narrative in its entirety is that she really enjoys telling stories. They are vivid and full of energy and use many strategies discussed previously to engage and draw the audience in. I hope the excerpts provided in this chapter have reflected these characteristics as well as provide some insights into the experience of black and ethnic minority nurse academics within the higher education sector.

References

Bamberg M G, and Andrews M (Eds) (2004) Considering Counter-Narratives: Narrating, Resisting, Making Sense. Amsterdam & Philadelphia: John Benjamins.

Beard, M (2018) Women and Power: A Manifesto. London: Profile Books.

Bhopal K, and Chapman T K (2019) International minority ethnic academics at predominantly white institutions. *British Journal of Sociology of Education*, 40(1), pp. 98–113.

Bhopal K (2010) Asian Women in Higher Education: Shared Communities. Stoke on Trent: Trentham.

Bhopal, K (2014) The experience of BME academics in higher education: Aspirations in the face of inequality. Leadership Foundation for Higher Education. Available at: www.advance-he.ac.uk/knowledge-hub/experience-bme-academics-higher-education-aspirationsface-inequality. Accessed: July 20, 2022.

Bhopal, K (2015) The Experience of Black and Minority Ethnic Academics in Higher Education: A Comparative Study of the Unequal Academy. London: Routledge Taylor & Francis Group.

Bhopal K, Brown H and Jackson J (2016) BME academic flight from UK to overseas higher education: aspects of marginalisation and exclusion. British Educational Research Journal, 42(2) pp. 240–257. doi: 10.1002/berj.3204

Bhopal K and Preston J (eds) (2012) Intersectionality and "Race" in Education. London: Routledge Taylor & Francis Group.

Bhui K, Nazroo J, Francis J, Halvorsrud K, and Rhodes K (2018) *The Impact of Racism on Mental Health: The Synergi Collaborative Centre.* Available at: https://synergicollaborativecentre.co.uk/wp-content/uploads/2017/11/The-impact-of-racism-on-mental-health-briefing-paper-1.pdf. Accessed: May 23 2021

Bonilla-Silva E (2014) Racism without Racist: Color-blind Racism and the Persistence of Racial Inequality in America (4th edn). Rowman & Littlefield Publishers, Incorporated. ISBN: 9781442220546

Charmaz, K (2006) Constructing Grounded Theory. Thousand Oaks, CA: Sage.

Cussins C M (1998) 'Ontological choreography: agency for women patients in an infertility clinic' in M Berg and S Mol (eds) Differences in Medicines: Unraveling Practices Techniques and Bodies. Durham, NC: Duke University Press, pp. 166–201.

Czarniawska B (2010) The uses of narratology in social and policy studies. Critical Policy Studies, 4, pp. 58–76. Quote is from Page 65

Delgado, R and Stefancic, J (1993) Critical race theory: an annotated bibliography. Virginia Law Review, 79(2), pp. 461–516. doi:10.2307/1073418

Delgado R and Stefancic J (2017) Critical Race Theory: An Introduction (3rd edn). New York: NYU Press. ISBN 147980276X, 9781479802760

Dentith S (1995) Bakhtinian Thought: An Introductory Reader. New York: Routledge.

DiAngelo, R (2018) White Fragility: Why It's So Hard for White People to Talk About Racism. US Penguin.

Equality and Human Rights Commission (2019) Tackling Racial Harassment: Universities Challenged. Available at: Tackling racial harassment: universities challenged | Equality and Human Rights Commission (equalityhumanrights.com). Accessed: July 20, 2022.

Freeman M (2002) 'The presence of what is missing: memory: poetry and the ride home' in R J Pellegrini and T R Sarbin (eds) Critical Incident Narratives in the Development of Men's lives. New York: Haworth Clinical Practice Press, pp. 165–176.

Frank A (1995) The Wounded Storyteller. Chicago, IL: University of Chicago Press.

Gee, J P (2011) An Introduction to Discourse Analysis: Theory and Method (3rd edn). London: Routledge.

Gee, J P (2014) How to Do Discourse Analysis (2nd edn). London: Routledge.

Goffman E (1974). Frame Analysis. An Essay on the Organisation of Experience. Cambridge, MA: Harvard University Pressing.

Harre R and van Langenhove L (eds) (1999) Positioning Theory. Malden: Blackwell.

Hill, P H and Bilge S (2016) Intersectionality. Cambridge: Politybooks.

Holder A M B M, Jackson M A, and Ponterotto J G (2015) Racial Microaggression Experiences and Coping Strategies of Black Women in Corporate Leadership. Qualitative Psychology American Psychological Association, 2(2), pp. 164–180.

Jensen, R (2021) Getting radical: Feminism, patriarchy, and the sexual-exploitation industries. Dignity: A Journal of Analysis of Exploitation and Violence, 6(2), Article 6. doi: 10.23860/dignity.2021.06.02.06

Khan M S, Lakha F, Tan M M J, Singh S R, Quek R Y C, Han E, Tan S M, Haldane V, Gea-Sánchez M, and Legido-Quigley H (2019) More talk than action: gender and ethnic diversity in leading public health universities. Lancet, 9(393(10171)), pp. 594–600. doi: 10.1016/S0140-6736(18)32609-6

Keashly L and Neuman J H (2010) Faculty Experiences with Bullying in Higher Education – Causes, Consequences, and Management. Available at: http://www.ccas.net/files/ADVANCE/Keashly_Bullying.pdf. Accessed: May 18, 2022.

Langellier K M (2001) '"You're marked": Breast cancer, tattoo and the narrative performance of identity' in Brockmeier and D Carbaugh (eds) Narrative Identity: Studies in Autobiographical, Self and Culture (pp. 145–184). Amsterdam & Philadelphia: John Benjamins.

Neuman J H and Baron R A (2005) 'Aggression in the workplace: A social psychological perspective' in S Fox and P E Spector (eds) Counterproductive Work Behavior: Investigations of Actors and Targets (pp. 13–40). Washington, DC: American Psychological Association.

Paradies Y, Ben J, Denson N, Elias A, Priest N, Pieterse A, Gupta A, Kelaher M, and Gee G. (2015) Racism as a determinant of health: A systematic review and meta-analysis. PLoS One. doi: 10.1371/journal.pone.0138511

Polanco-Roman L, Danies A, and Anglin D M (2016) Racial discrimination as race-based trauma, coping strategies and dissociative symptoms among emerging adults. Psychological Trauma, 8(5), 609–617. doi: 10.1037/tra0000125

Riessman C K (1993) Narrative Analysis. Newbury Park, CA: Sage.

Riessman C K (2008) Narrative Methods for the Human Sciences. London: Sage.

Riessman C K (2016) 'What's different about narrative inquiry? Cases, categories and context' in Silverman D (ed) Qualitative Research (4th edn, pp. 363–378). London: Sage.

Rollock N (2019) Staying Power: The Career Experiences and Strategies of UK Black FEMALE PROFESsors. University and College Union (UCU).

Sue D W (2010) Microaggressions in Everyday Life: Race, Gender, and Sexual Orientation. John Wiley & Sons Inc.

Sue D W, Alsaidi S, Awad, M N, Glaeser, E, Calle, C Z, and Mendez N (2019) Disarming racial microaggressions: Microintervention strategies for targets, White allies, and bystanders. American Psychologist, 74(1), pp. 128–142. https://doi.org/10.1037/amp0000296

Sue D W, Capodilupo C M, and Holder A M B (2007) Racial microaggressions in the life experience of Black Americans. Professional Psychology: Research and Practice, 39(3), pp. 329–336. https://doi.org/10.1037/0735-7028.39.3.329

Universities UK (UUK) (2020) Tackling Racial Harassment in Higher Education. Available at: tackling-racial-harassment-in-higher-education.pdf (universitiesuk.ac.uk). Accessed: July 20, 2022.

Williams M (2020) Managing Microaggressions: Addressing Everyday Racism in Therapeutic Spaces. New York. Oxford University Press.

Williams M T and Sharif N (2021) Racial allyship: novel measurement and new insights. New Ideas in Psychology, 62, p. 100865. https://doi.org/10.1016/j.newideapsych.2021.100865

Wolfson N (1989) 'The conversational historic present' in Linx, n°20. Analyse grammaticale des corpus oraux (pp. 135–151). Available at: https://www.persee.fr/doc/linx_0246-8743_1989_num_20_1_1125 https://doi.org/10.3406/linx.1989.1125. Accessed: June 12, 2022.

8 Racism in nursing

The more things change, the more they stay the same

Petula Gordon

The NHS

The National Health Service (NHS) is a publicly funded health care organisation that was set up in 1948 (Gov.UK, 2016). It was born out of an ideal that good health care should be available to all regardless of means. Treatment is free at the point of use for people resident in the United Kingdom (UK) (Gov. UK, 2016). The NHS constitution which was created to protect the NHS, stipulates that free high-quality care should be at its core, and core values shape an organisation's culture (LinkedIn, 2015). The stated values of the NHS are: Respect and dignity for all individuals; Commitment to quality of care, learning from mistakes; Compassion, where staff are humane to those being served and also to the people they work alongside; Improving lives through the measures put in place to ensure the health and well-being of all; Working together for patients where the needs of patients and communities come first; Everyone counts, where no-one is excluded and resources are used for the benefit of all (Gov.UK, 2016). The aim of the NHS should be the promotion of health which is rooted in shared values of equality, sustainability and the common good (Bambra et al., 2005); however, the period after the Second World War saw a rise in racism (Carter, 2002; Cregan, 2010; Vonderbeck and Worth, 2015) following a call from the British government for black people from the commonwealth countries to help rebuild post-war Britain (Henry, 1985). Nurses from the British colonies were recruited into roles that were difficult to recruit to, jobs that the indigenous people did not want to do such as working in mental health and care of the elderly (Ali et al., 2013). Ali et al. (2013) argue that having a diverse workforce was often considered a problem by the health service in the 1960s. John (2015) asserts that receiving racial abuse was not unusual for black nurses when tending to patients in the 1960s. Words such as '*Get your filthy black hands off me*', or '*go and get a white nurse to attend to me and go back to where you came from*' (John, 2015, p. 2) were commonplace. He also shares that there were others in the workplace who would orchestrate situations to put black nurses in trouble with nursing supervisors. Sue (2010) and Lais (2019) describe the experiences John (2015) cites, as micro-aggressions in which

DOI: 10.4324/9781003269915-8

victims are subjected to hostile and negative messages, verbal and non-verbal slights. Micro-aggressions are targeted at people based solely on membership of their marginalised group which can have a powerful effect on individuals. The concept of micro-aggressions will be examined later in this chapter.

Today, the NHS is in crisis (Nursing and Midwifery Council (NMC), 2017). Figures published in July 2017 demonstrated that for the first time in its history, the number of UK nurses leaving the NHS exceeded the number of nurses joining (NMC, 2017). The number joining had fallen markedly from 10,178 to 1,107 between October 2016 and September 2017, representing a decrease of 89% in 12 months. Nurses and midwives were leaving the nurse register before the age of retirement with a notable increase in those under the age of 40 leaving the NHS (NMC, 2017). The staff shortfall was attributed, in part, to Black and Minority Ethnic (BME) nurses leaving the NHS due to being disadvantaged regarding access to professional development opportunities as they were less likely to be selected to attend such programmes (Kline and Prabhu, 2015). Jones (2000) argues that the first generation of health workers from overseas experienced discrimination around training and career opportunities which has impacted negatively on the recruitment of the second generation. The NHS was built on a diverse workforce and continues to depend on a diverse workforce (Jones-Berry, 2017) yet a report by the Workforce Race Equality Standard (WRES) reports that it is apparent BME nurses and midwives are severely and persistently disadvantaged in the workplace which in turn has led to an acute shortage of qualified health professionals (Nadeem, 2019). Discrimination against BME staff has been an ongoing concern within the NHS for many years (Kline, 2014; Archibong and Darr, 2010). With the Chief Executive Officer (CEO) of the NMC describing it as a disgrace, reports suggest that there had been a rise in discrimination against BME staff from 13.8% to 15% in the year from 2018 to 2019 (NHS WRES, 2019; The Royal College of Nursing [RCN], 2019). This contrasts with the experiences of white staff in the NHS where discrimination is just 6.6% (NHS WRES, 2019).

Staff loss contributed to the 11,400 nurse and midwife shortfall in 2017, costing the NHS up to £2.4 billion (Wilson, 2018) for utilising agency nurses to fill the gaps in both the hospitals and the community. Projected figures suggested that there would be a nurse shortfall of 42,000 in 2020 if steps were not taken to offset the shortage. On 31 December 2021, data showed that there was a vacancy rate of 39,652 for registered nurses (NHS Digital, 2022). As a black woman nurse specialist working for the NHS, I was concerned with inequitable practices and the resultant staff losses that I observed within the NHS. Reports suggested that discrimination was evident with levels notably high for black employees and were highest amongst black nurses (Merrifield, 2015). When deciding on a career path, the core values of the NHS were a factor for me choosing to work for the organisation, coupled with the expectation that those entering the nursing profession shared the same beliefs. However, observing staff in action in their various roles, I came to a different understanding which presented a different picture. Behaviours fell short of the NHS's core values with discriminatory practices being an ongoing concern regarding black nurses accessing training and development programmes compared to their white peers.

According to the Equality and Human Rights Commission (EHRC, 2019), there are three types of discrimination: direct, indirect and discrimination arising from disability. Direct discrimination pertains to treating someone with a protected characteristic less favourably than someone without a protected characteristic, for instance, refusing a student entry to education because of their characteristic (Equal Opportunities Commission [EOC], 2021). This characteristic could refer to age, religion, gender, race and so forth. Indirect discrimination is said to have occurred when a policy may place an individual at a disadvantage in the workplace. For instance, in the case of religion, a person who has to work on a day that they would be attending church would be classed as being discriminated against indirectly (EHRC, 2019). Anyone who has a disability and is treated unfavourably as a result is said to have been discriminated against (EOC, 2021).

I conducted my doctoral research to ascertain the NHS's current position. I asked whether the culture of the NHS was prejudiced or racist or if it could be both prejudiced and racist. In order to locate my research, I examined the concepts of discrimination as defined earlier and also looked at prejudice and racism. I examine each concept in turn in the following sections.

Prejudice and discrimination

Prejudice is defined as

A favourable or unfavourable preconceived feeling or opinion formed without knowledge, reason, or thought, that prevents objective consideration of person, group, or thing.

(Bell, 2013)

Allport (1954, p. 9) argues that prejudice is a premature judgment that resists facts and ignores truth and honesty and asserts that ethnic prejudice is an antipathy based upon a faulty and inflexible generalisation. Worchel et al. (1998) suggest that prejudice is a negative attitude that is unjustified and exists solely because of a persons' membership of that group. Brown (1995) agrees with Allport (1954) and Worchel et al. (1998) asserting that prejudice can be understood as the derogatory belief and hostile behaviour towards membership of a group based solely on their membership of that group. For example, gender which is a source of prejudice (Dovidio and Gaertner, 2010) otherwise known as sexism (BBC Bitesize, 2020) occurs when an individual is treated differently because of their sex or gender (Equality Hub, 2016). Both men and women can be victims of sexism but it mainly affects women (BBC Bitesize, 2020). There are individuals who are subject to prejudices on several fronts if for instance they are of colour and female (Bell and Mahmood, 2016) (see literature on intersectionality).

Having looked at discrimination and prejudice, the next section examines racism.

Racism

The Human Rights Act 2010 sets out the fundamental rights and freedoms that everyone in the UK is entitled to (Human Rights Act, 2010). The act exists by virtue of the fact that basic rights belong to humans (Equality Hub, 2016). These rights embody key values in society, values such as fairness, equality, dignity and respect (Equality Hub, 2016).[1]

Traditionally, racism has been defined as the unfair and negative treatment towards a particular group of people based on their ethnicity or race (Fish and Syed, 2019). This definition has been criticised for being limited as it fails to take into account the factors that are important in understanding racism, factors such as history, power and privilege (Cole and Harper, 2017). Racism has thus been defined as

> *A system of power entwined with practices and beliefs that produce and maintain an ethnic and racial hierarchy. The preservation of this ethnic and racial hierarchy in turn, leads to the superiority, power, and privilege of some, and the oppression of others.*
>
> (Fish and Syed, 2019, p. 5)

Hilliard (1992) argues that racism has been described by 'whiteness' scholars as a system that comprises political, economic, social, actions, beliefs and cultural structures that systematically perpetuate unequal distributions of resources, power and privileges between white people and people of colour (POC). Although the term 'people of colour' is used in this chapter, it is not an uncontested term as there is the argument that 'white' is also a colour (Lamuye, 2017). However, for the purposes of this chapter, the term POC is used to facilitate understanding.

Being white accrues privilege and status (Fine, 1997). White privilege refers to the unearned benefits white people receive just for being part of the dominant group (Bell, 2013; Home Office, 1999). Put another way, white people are the beneficiaries to the unequal distribution whilst POC are disadvantaged (Frankenberg, 1993; Hilliard, 1992). A specific dimension of racism is "whiteness" as a social process which is inseparable from systems of injustice (DiAngelo, 2011). Whiteness is purported to be the means by which white people elevate themselves over POC (Home Office, 1999; Mcintosh, 1989). Whiteness has been defined as multi-dimensional and is described by Frankenberg

> *Whiteness is a location of structural advantage, of race privilege. Second, it is a 'standpoint,' a place from which White people look at*

ourselves, at others, and at society. Third, 'Whiteness' refers to a set of
cultural practices that are usually unmarked and unnamed.

(Frankenberg, 1993, p. 1)

Faruqui, who became Australia's first Muslim woman senator, argued in her first Senate speech that racism is normalised by the media and politicians (Knaus, 2018) supporting the argument of Hilliard (1992) and Frankenberg (1993) that power and privilege are features of racism. Faruqui argued that whilst politicians display public solidarity in condemning the most blatant racism, this can be in fact a cover for their role in creating and stirring up racial divisions. This occurs in the case of institutional racism where the be-havioural norms of individuals or informal social groups are supported by racist thinking and the instigation of active racism (Home Office, 1999). The institutional aspect of racism is the result of its construction within an or-ganisation, having historical roots and being allowed to remain as it goes unchallenged and is not questioned (DiAngelo, 2011). The effect of this is that institutional racism becomes embedded within an organisation, impact-ing POC negatively as deep rooted structures are allowed to remain where POC constantly face stigma and marginalisation when accessing health care and public services, including the justice system, prison service and immigra-tion system (Jones, 1997; Lais, 2019). This is perpetuated by the policies, practices, procedures and the culture of an organisation which largely ex-cludes POC from having a voice and from benefitting from opportunities and resources (Crenshaw et al., 1996). These actions serve to reinforce individual attitudes and prejudices, with POC being marginalised, isolated and stigma-tised culminating in sustained trauma.

Having looked at the concepts of prejudice and racism during my doctoral study, and based on the understanding of both concepts, I viewed the NHS through the lens of racism being aware of the difference between prejudice and racism (Andrews, 2015). Focusing on individual prejudice avoids dealing with the endemic systematic racism which results in significant inequalities (Andrews, 2015). Robin DiAngelo (2011), who is a white woman, asserts that mainstream definitions of racism are usually some variation of individ-ual race prejudice which can be held by anyone, but in reality, racism is about social processes.

My personal experience

One of the drivers for undertaking my research was my experience as a black woman working within the NHS. Sultana (2007) argues that for the researcher to engage in ethical research, it is critical that s/he pays attention to positionality, reflexivity, the production of knowledge and the power rela-tions that are characteristic of research processes (Sultana, 2007).

Personal experiences are real and subjective therefore I acknowledge that there is researcher bias which Mehra (2002) asserts is inevitable when conducting research. Some may see my subjectivity as self-indulgent but Bravette (1997) would argue that as a nurse educator and a leader, I am a role model for others. Being objective when having an experience is said by the philosopher Renee Descartes to be impossible and therefore asserts that we know knowledge with certainty through our ability to think (Burns, 2001). In other words, reality exists because we observe it. Moustakas (1994) proffers that the researcher writes about their own experience and the situations that have influenced their research. Furthermore, Hall (2005) argues that self-narratives are found in every culture and are a uniquely human way of understanding the world.

I begin by recounting an experience I had when I secured my first senior role as lead nurse for the Tuberculosis (TB) service in an area of the UK which at the time had the highest rates of TB. I was a standalone practitioner which meant I ran the service single handedly. I was specifically recruited for this temporary role even though I had no prior experience of this area of medicine. I forged ahead however and quickly learned the role. I moved from novice to expert through developing skills and a sound educational base along with the experience of working with the client group (Benner, 1982). I achieved this with the aid of key literature, policies and protocols and the help of key staff to assist me e.g. respiratory consultants, specialist nurses and health advocates who acted as translators for those patients who did not have English as a first language.

With increasing knowledge, I achieved well against the key performance indicators i.e. I achieved 89% TB treatment completion rates against the national and global performance target of 85% (TB Facts, 2018). Three months into the role, the job was advertised nationally. Believing my experience was insufficient, I did not apply. A white male nurse who had a few years' experience within the field was appointed to the permanent position. After his appointment, I was taken on substantively as his deputy. Shortly after my appointment, he told me that I could not access further training as I had 'had my quota of training' despite the fact I was new to the field and needed the training in order to provide the patients with quality care based on the best available evidence (RCN, 2018). My black colleague was also not allowed to access training courses in contrast to white staff members who were able to undertake training as part of their development. I eventually left that organisation.

I subsequently worked in another NHS organisation where I had a similar experience. I was denied training and told I would have to wait until the following year to access it despite training funds being available. Staffing was not an issue as the team was fully staffed and two white staff members had declined training. Staffing however was used as the excuse as to why I could not pursue a course even though the training would have mainly been conducted online via the internet. I had reached the top of my nursing band, my pay was capped and there was no place for me to progress further, so I was unable to improve further to serve the patients better.

The RCN (2018) refers to the experiences I cite as workplace incivility which is defined as the condition where low intensity behaviour occurs with the ambiguous intent to cause harm. Rather than foster an inclusive workforce where staff are supported to perform well, workplace incivility works against the targeted staff and leads to a toxic culture, a situation which characterises the culture of some workplaces (RCN, 2018). I wanted to develop my skills as a practitioner and avoid stagnation in order to remain motivated but as this was not allowed, I left the organisation shortly after and worked as an independent contractor.

As a reflexive practitioner, I try to make sense of my experiences in the workplace so that the learning can be applied to practice which in turn benefits the patients. Chiavaroli and Trumble (2018) argue that exercising phronesis in matters such as these would prove beneficial to the functioning of organisations as it enables, in this case the practitioner, to use practical wisdom in determining what action to take. Kinsella and Pitman (2012) state that:

> *Phronesis is an intellectual virtue that implies ethics. It involves deliberation that is based on values, concerned with practical judgment and informed by reflection. It is pragmatic, variable, context dependent and oriented towards action.*
>
> (Kinsella and Pitman, 2012, p. 2)

In exercising practical wisdom, I adopted the concepts from Kolb's (1984) learning cycle in which I reflected on each experience which Kolb (1984) refers to as having a concrete experience. From the experiences, I was drawing conclusions or what Kolb (1984) refers to as abstract conceptualisations where I was making sense of what was happening, reflecting on what I had done and what I already knew. I then moved onto the final stage of Kolb's (1984) learning cycle which was to act in order to address the situation in question. I did so by requesting a meeting with the manager of the first organisation that I cite.

I expressed my concerns to the manager in a professional manner to *challenge while keeping relationships intact* (Naylor, 2008, p. 5). Without warning, this resulted in a letter summoning me to a disciplinary meeting whilst on annual leave which naturally upset the time I was taking away from the workplace to renew my energy. Being subject to a disciplinary hearing was not something I had faced in all my years of nursing. The usual procedure in bringing a disciplinary against a staff member was not followed as it is a process that progresses through stages if there is no improvement in whatever the situation may be. The first stage is a verbal warning, followed by a written warning then a disciplinary meeting (Employment Law Clinic, 2018). This did not happen in my case, I was summoned directly to a disciplinary meeting for voicing my concerns. NHS England (2016) argue that too many NHS organisations move to a formal investigation as the default position without even considering whether it is a necessary course of action. It is situations like this why many nurses are of the belief that equality in the NHS is a myth (Keogh, 2019). Atewologun and Singh (2010) argue that black professionals often have to oppose the stereotypes that they encounter in those cultures that fail to value diversity. It has been said that the system is not set up for black people, their talent and skills are not valued. In the situations I have described, as a reflexive practitioner, the action I took was necessary for the benefit and the functioning of the organisation (Chiavaroli and Trumble, 2018). The alternative would be to do nothing whilst discriminatory practices go unchallenged and work relations deteriorate further.

DiAngelo (2018) refers to the reaction to the experience I cite as 'white fragility' which occurs when white people are protected against race-based stress with a lowered ability to tolerate racial stress. For instance, if the assumptions white people hold about race are challenged, the reaction becomes defensive and counterproductive and acts as a means of maintaining racial inequality through behaviours such as anger, guilt, fear, aversion, argument and walking away from the stress inducing situation (Allen, 2001; DiAngelo, 2018). DiAngelo, a former professor and lecturer who works as a facilitator and a consultant, is hired by organisations to look at the recruitment of BME staff and to uncover why they fail to stay in organisations. She found that in instances of racial discrimination when BME people challenged white people, this resulted in outrage at the suggestion of them being racist. Although DiAngelo's (2018) remit is to make visible the racist assumptions held about BME people which occurs as a result of the conditioning through living in a white supremist culture, the responses that resulted when questioned or named, yielded the same predictable responses which was that of outrage. DiAngelo (2018) is asked to deliver workshops to help the staff see their racism but when she helps them see the racism, she is met with hostility, anger, argument, silence, defence, withdrawal. In other words, white fragility erupts and functions to protect racial inequality.

The point is illustrated when during one of her workshops she states:

> *I have just presented a definition of racism that includes the acknowledgment that whites hold social and institutional power over people of colour. A white man is pounding his fist on the table. His face is red and he is furious. As he pounds he yells, "White people have been discriminated against for 25 years! A white person can't get a job anymore!" I look around the room and see 40 employed people, all white. There are no people of colour in this workplace.*
>
> (DiAngelo, 2011, pp. 54–70)

Racism as a system is concealed and protected due to the widespread understanding that to be racist requires conscious intent, an understanding that practically exempts all white people with some not wishing to be seen as racist (Kivel, 2017). This is due in part to the post-civil rights era where people have been taught that racists are mean with an intentional dislike for others based on their race, including being intentionally hurtful and consciously prejudiced (Kivel, 2017). Similar to Kivel's (2017) argument, Hefferman (2014) argues that people are compelled to develop and protect a positive image of self. To deny that racism exists is known as the new racism as it pertains to ignoring or turning a blind eye to a vice that actually exists (Lee Hall, 2016). In America, it is said that most white people choose to deny that racism exist as a cover to avoid the fear and negative publicity that is associated with being seen to support it (Lee Hall, 2016).

During my learning journey as a research student, I found it profound to reflect on 'white fragility' as one of many means by which racial inequality is perpetuated and equilibrium maintained in society. My research was needed because the omission of the experiences and perspectives of black nurses regarding their professional development in the NHS has consequences (Watson-Druee, 2009). Ignoring the voice and experiences of the small group of black women practitioners who have achieved, creates a blockage for growth and development through a lack of awareness for a younger generation (Kline, 2014). Whilst the focus of my research was on BME nurses, I acknowledge that there are inequalities among other marginalised groups such as gay/transgender or disabled people but as the literature alludes to, black people are oppressed and do not have any adaptions and existing laws do not always protect them. Instead, they are silenced and told that they are 'playing the race card' when they try to voice concerns (Hirsch, 2020). It was my aim to help the reader to understand the phenomenon of racism and its impact on health that may otherwise be difficult to understand or interpret (Eisner, 1991). I was interested in the nurses' accounts of their own experiences and points of view.

Research methodology and design

I conducted a review of the literature to inform my project in order to critically appraise how different researchers had addressed the issues raised. This was to gain insight to the knowledge relevant to my project. The primary purpose of the review was to uncover why discriminatory practices exist, how they are perpetuated and how the experience of BME nurses could be improved when it came to accessing training and professional development activities within the NHS.

Bacharach (1989) asserts that theories are used in research to explain and analyse phenomena under investigation. Critical race theory (CRT) was chosen to guide my inquiry. CRT is a theoretical framework that is used to explore society and culture in relation to law, race and power and is used to look at different forms of oppression (Yosso, 2005). CRT was used as a method in my project to critique the literature and the findings i.e. the role of race and racism that maintains the status-quo of racism (Huber, 2008). CRT emerged in the 1970s in the United States of America (USA) in response to the slow rate at which the racial equality laws were changing (Cole, 2007; Crenshaw et al., 1996). Despite civil laws which stipulate that all human beings living in society are entitled to be free from discrimination and lead happy and healthy lives, free from people and organisational intrusion and unwarranted persecution (Cole, 2007), CRT proposes that societal racism or white supremacy in which white people are privileged, is maintained over time with the law being seen as a contributor to oppression (Crenshaw et al., 1996). Prejudicial attitudes are institutionalised into laws and structures that favour one race over the other, structures that are created to set up POC to fail through keeping them in oppressive states thereby disempowering them (Crenshaw, 1988).

Utley (2016) contends that race which is socially constructed as opposed to being biologically grounded and natural, acts as a means to perpetuate the interest of the white population who constructed it. In relation to CRT, Utley (2016) agrees with Crenshaw et al. (1996) and asserts that legal structures and policies which are biased against POC, contribute to the inequality between the 'races' through keeping the so called minority groups impoverished, creating the conditions for criminality to arise in a bid to survive. Utley (2016) further contends that white people create this difference to ensure an elitist structure is maintained through the social and economic differences they create in labour markets and politics and have no interest in doing away with these practices because they benefit them. Crenshaw (1988) argues that the status quo of oppression is further strengthened as merely acknowledging America's history of racism, is seen to be disparaging and unpatriotic and has seen activists such as those in the civil rights movement targeted, placed under surveillance and disrupted by law enforcement agencies such as the Federal Bureau of Investigation (FBI). There appears to be a disconnect however as amongst the FBI's role, one of its top priorities is ostensibly to protect the civil rights of people occupying American territory whether they are citizens or non-citizens (FBI, 2016).

Other forces that disempower black people and maintain oppressive and elitist structures include actions such as on-going assassinations which were prevalent during the civil rights movement in the USA when those who stood up for the rights of black people became assassination targets (McCalla, 2011).

Yosso (2005) a professor of education, uses CRT through the lens of a community cultural wealth model to examine POC, as opposed to the traditional deficit model of cultural capital in which POC are viewed as being impoverished and disadvantaged. Her work examines their individual and shared experiences of discrimination and marginalisation in education. Using counter stories, Yosso (2005) brought to the fore, the knowledge, skills and abilities that the POC possess and challenged the deficit model of CRT. She did this by focusing on cultural wealth which provides learning in the range of cultural knowledge, skills and abilities that socially marginalised groups possess which are often not acknowledged and go unrecognised. Yosso (2005) argues that theory enables the generation of knowledge, some of which have been kept from POC because entry into some professions and academia has been denied. Therefore, because they have been barred from certain discourses, there is an urgent need for POC to occupy the theorising space that is afforded to white men and women (Anzaldúa, 1990).

The question asked concerning the epistemology or the sources of knowledge is "whose knowledge counts and whose knowledge is discounted?" (Delgado-Bernal, 1998, 2002; Ladson-Billings and Tate, 2000). López (2001) argues that race and racism have shaped the epistemological debate and those individuals who are born into a privileged society are deemed to have knowledge that is of capital value to a hierarchical society. For those who have not been born into a privileged society, social mobility may be achieved through formal education in which the knowledge of the middle and upper classes is accessed (Bourdieu and Passeron, 1990). Based on the strategies that are used to disenfranchise, it is assumed that POC are deficient in the social and cultural capital required for social mobility. In response to the theories and assumptions held about POC, Anzaldúa (1990) states

> *If we have been gagged and disempowered by theories, we can also be loosened and empowered by theories.*
>
> (Anzaldúa, 1990, p. 26)

The argument being put forward is that the voices and presence of POC can be valued through other sources of knowledge such as outsider knowledge. Disempowerment is the means by which hierarchical society is reproduced, maintained and interpreted to be the reason why POC have significantly lower outcomes academically and socially when compared to white people (Bourdieu and Passeron, 1990). In other words, through deliberate means, POC are limited in being able to change social reality by social, political and cultural domination.

Data collection

My research question sought to address how to extend and improve knowledge of the experiences of BME nurses when seeking to access training and development programmes within the NHS. A questionnaire survey, interviews and my reflective journal were the methods I used to collect data from two NHS Trusts. The questionnaire was used as a means of exploring how nurses access professional development opportunities so that the extent of the issue being investigated could be ascertained. Sofaer (1999) argues that data enhances understanding of the context of events as well as the events themselves. Individual interviews were also used in my study in order to enable participants to describe their experience in-depth, thereby providing more meaningful explanations (Tahan and Sminkey, 2012). Semi structured interviews with scripted questions were compiled to allow for the flexibility to probe the participants' answers (Laverack, 2005). I commenced a reflective journal at the start of my project as a learning tool and a means of being transparent where my experiences, thoughts, feelings and opinions would be visible (Ortlipp, 2008). I employed Interpretative Phenomenological Analysis (IPA) as a methodology for my study which I will expand on later. Flowers et al. (2005) recommend for researchers engaging in IPA, that through making notes and looking back over the course of their learning journey, they should be able to chart their development. My sample population included nurses from all nationalities so that I could gain a full picture of what was happening in practice as it was felt that the study could have wider implications for those employed in the NHS, where discriminatory practices could transcend a range of ethnic groups. The inclusion criteria were that the nurses had to be fully trained, working within the NHS or having previously worked in the NHS. Their job banding (grades) had to be from 5 to 9, occupying roles such as staff nurses, sisters/charge nurses or senior nurses. The exclusion criterion for the project was untrained nurses. The plan was to circulate survey questionnaires to at least 100 nurse participants to try and obtain a representative sample and to obtain 12 to 15 participants for the interviews. The actual number of survey questionnaires that I analysed was 40 and I interviewed 12 participants of those who also took part in the survey.

Being influenced by a post positivist perspective, I chose to adopt a constructivist stance as my research sought to explore the experiences of the participants. It sought to understand the social world from their standpoint and the meaning they attributed to the context in which events that have meaning, occurred (Letts et al., 2007). This approach is in contrast to a positivist stance generally understood as an assumption that there is a single reality or truth which exists independently of any consciousness (Crotty, 1998; Denzin and Lincoln, 2011).

I sought a methodological framework where emphasis was on a conscious knowledge enabling the research participants to convey what was perceived, sensed and known, based on their experience (Moustakas, 1994). Smith and Osborn (2015) argue that this type of approach enables exploration of the participants' lived experience and what the experiences mean to them. As a black woman nurse practitioner with experience of the phenomenon under investigation, a methodological framework was sought which took account of my own assumptions and philosophical values.

Methodology

I utilised IPA as it is *a philosophy and research method that studies experienced events and objects using the senses* (Bell, 2013). It is a qualitative research approach which assumes that there is an essence to shared experience (Letts, 2003; Marshall and Rossman, 2006). I used IPA to analyse the interview data as it places emphasis on the researcher being involved in the process of interpretation (Smith and Osborn, 2015). It seeks to describe in precise detail, a phenomenon that is experienced by the individual and focuses on the subjective experiences of the individual (Smith and Osborn, 2015). IPA was deemed an appropriate framework for my project as it fitted with the research aim in which I sought to gain an insight into the research participants' experiences in order to understand the phenomenon of a lived experience (Letts, 2003). I needed a research approach that would enable engagement with the research question at an idiographic level or, put another way, an individual or unique level (Flowers et al., 2005).

Findings

The findings from my research indicated that BME nurses still faced discrimination when attempting to access training and development programmes with black nurses being more disadvantaged than other marginalised nurses. The findings from the survey questionnaires and interviews are demonstrated below.

Surveys

Forty participants took part in the questionnaire survey. Twenty-four of the nurse participants identified as BME, eight identified as British and six identified as white British. Of the 40 respondents, 36 reported that there was a culture of training and development within their organisation and that they were able to access training programmes. Those participants who were able to access training reported a good working relationship with their manager. There was a correlation between those nurses who were able to access training, with feeling respected, being valued as a member of the team and being part of the decision-making process.

I selected 12 of the 40 survey participants to invite to take part in the interviews as the particular answers they provided in the questionnaires prompted further interest and required deeper probing. The interviews are discussed in the next section.

Interviews

The 12 nurses who took part in the interviews were from a BME background with ages ranging from 40 to 70, having a total of 234 years of nursing experience between them. The highest nursing band achieved within the participant group was a band 7, registered nurse bands range from 5 to 9. Being able to interview the nurses meant I could probe further especially if information included in the questionnaires demonstrated that further exploration was required.

I have included some excerpts below from the interview. All names have been changed to protect the identity of the participants.

The following participant related her experience when asked whether she thought there was equality amongst all staff when trying to access training courses:

> *It's unfortunate that when you're talking about training and development and then when you are talking about race and equality and diversity, you somehow... I just realised at the beginning of the interview, I was really talking quite heatedly about experiences that I went through. So when you say training, when you say professional development, then race somehow rears its nasty head in there. It's very difficult to separate sometimes, so I'm sorry about that.*
>
> (Abigail, interviewee 6)

When I asked another participant the same question she said:

> *When they talk about equality, they talk about erm, equity and all these things but it's just erm, written on the paper but they don't apply that. You do ask for the training, they will ask you a few things, so many things to complete. But when a Caucasian comes, they don't even need to complete what they've been asked for, they just put them on that training straight away, ...obviously if you are from, if you are a different, erm, erm, let's just say if you are a black person like I am.*
>
> (Esther, interviewee 7)

Another participant was asked the same question as to whether there was equality across all ethnic groups, to which she replied:

> *No way! I believe they are not treated fairly. First of all, wherever there is a minority, there'll be some form of inequality because there will be a lack of support and lack of understanding of the staff culture.*
>
> (Dinah, interviewee 8)

What I have presented here is a small sample of the data from the interviews, but the general consensus among the participants was that racism is being used as a means of preventing black nurses from reaching their full potential through a lack of non-mandatory training opportunities which was having a negative impact on the care that patients receive. The participants shared how racism/discriminatory practices adversely affected clinical practice. The following excerpt from one participant is presented as it encapsulates the feelings of most of the participants:

> *Because they ill-treat the workers, it's the patients in the end who bear the brunt because when an extra nurse or carer could be there to help wash the patient, feed the patient, they're not there, because they are probably off sick because they're overworked. People are lying in bed,*

sometimes people are ill, they can't feed themselves and they haven't touched it because they can't reach the food, they can't help themselves.
(Mary, interviewee 10)

Conclusion and recommendations

Tackling race inequalities within the NHS has been a longstanding problem. As black professionals occupy senior positions, the issues they face will make it difficult for organisations to retain talent (Atewologun and Singh 2010). As well as the NHS losing valuable staff, it limits the advancement of leadership potential for younger practitioners and perpetuates the status quo (Kline, 2014). Bhopal and Alibhai-Brown (2018) concur with John (2014) and Douglas (1995) in asserting that racism is structural and is woven into the very fabric of society, existing at all levels of society including higher educational institutions. According to Crenshaw (1988), racism is structured disadvantage where laws establish actual practices of exclusion and disadvantage. Despite the strategies put in place to combat the inequalities within the NHS e.g. organisational policies, diversity training and so forth, the evidence from the literature and data suggests that there have been no significant changes.

Whilst several contributory factors pertaining to discrimination emerged whilst undertaking my research, racism was a prominent feature according to the research data. The evidence suggests that racism persists because of the structures that are in place to maintain the status-quo. The literature demonstrated that racism is structural and underpins the operation of the NHS (Douglas, 1995; John, 2014) which implies that it operates along the same racist structures that is endemic in British society. In other words, those who hold a core belief that is very strong (racists in this case), despite being presented with evidence that works against that belief, will not accept it. The feeling that the evidence creates when brought to the fore is one of discomfort. This according to Owuor (2017) is attributed to white people expecting black people to carry the burden of proving that racism exists even though it is white people that mostly cause the discriminatory practices. Owuor (2017) asserts that when it is proven that racism exists, black people face the resultant backlash and are subjected to excuses.

My research findings indicate that change, with a focus on leadership, within the NHS is needed if it is to survive. The evidence points to the NHS needing a joined-up approach where individual nurses, NHS Trusts and government bodies work together to address the issues the findings raise. In order to address the findings, it is recommended that strategies are put in place such as NHS Trusts implementing stringent monitoring systems in relation to training that is outside the managerial remit of the specific clinical sector, whereby if discriminatory incidents concerned with professional development and training needs occur but are not addressed, they can be independently identified and those Trusts held to account. This would also include monitoring training access as per the public sector equality duty (EHRC, 2021) which stipulates that discrimination, harassment and victimisation is unlawful.

What appears to be lacking in the NHS is accountability for poor practice. The human resources/training departments of the NHS need to implement and oversee a system whereby not only mandatory courses are monitored but also a mandatory stringent monitoring system should be established to audit the personal and professional development of black nurses in particular. The department would also need to be held accountable if staff were not being developed. Through adopting these strategies, it is hoped that this process would elicit change as it is this change that will help black nurses survive and thrive in the NHS environment.

Note

1 This topic has been debated over centuries.

References

Agyemang, C., Bhopal, R. and Brujnzeels, M. (2005). 'Negro, Black, Black African, African Caribbean, African American or What? Labelling African origins populations in the health arena in the 21st century'*Journal of Epidemiology and Community Health*, 59, pp. 1014–1018. doi: 10.1136/Tech.2005.035964.

Ali, S., Burns, C. and Grant, L. (2013). 'Scaling the NHS's diversity problems', *Health Service Journal* [Online]. Available at: https://www.hsj.co.uk/leadership/scaling-the-nhss-diversity-problems/5065264.article (Accessed: 10 October 2017).

Allen, R.L. (2001). 'The globalization of white supremacy: Toward a critical discourse on the racialization of the world', *Educational Theory*, 51(4), pp. 467–485.

Allport, G. (1954). *The Nature of Prejudice*. 25th edn. Reading, MA: Addison-Wesley.

Andrews, K. (2015). 'Racism is still alive and well, 50 years after the UK's Race Relations Act', *The Guardian*, 8 December [Online]. Available at: https://www.theguardian.com/commentisfree/2015/dec/08/50-anniversary-race-relations-act-uk-prejudice-racism (Accessed: 11 August 2019).

Anzaldúa, G. (1990). *Making Face, Making Soul/Haciendo Caras. Creative and Critical Perspectives by Women of Color*. San Francisco, CA: Aunt Lute Book.

Archibong, U. and Darr, A. (2010). *The Involvement of Black and Minority Ethnic Staff in NHS Disciplinary Proceedings*. Bradford: University of Bradford.

Atewologun, D. and Singh, V. (2010). 'Challenging ethnic and gender identities,' *Equality, Diversity and Inclusion: An International Journal*, 29(4) [Online]. Available at: https://www.deepdyve.com/lp/emerald-publishing/challenging-ethnic-and-gender-identities-an-exploration-of-uk-black-INWbxiS0fi (Accessed: 21 August 2019).

Bacharach, S.B. (1989). 'Organizational theories: Some criteria for evaluation', *Academy of Management Review*, 14(4), pp. 496–515.

Bambra, C., Fox, D. and Scott-Samuel, A. (2005). 'Towards a politics of health', *Health Promotion International*, 20(2), pp. 187–193.

BBC. (2020). 'Theatre drops use of "outdated" term BAME', *BBC News*, 17 July [Online]. Available at: https://www.bbc.co.uk/news/uk-england-coventry-warwickshire-53446837 (Accessed: 20 July 2020).

BBC Bitesize. (2020). *Prejudice and Discrimination*. Available at: https://www.bbc.co.uk/bitesize/guides/zcb42hv/revision/2 (Accessed: 15 January 2020).

Bell, B. and Mahmood, S. (2016). 'What did the "strikers in saris" achieve?', *BBC News*, 10 September [Online]. Available at: https://www.bbc.co.uk/news/uk-england-london-37244466 (Accessed: 26 March 2020).

Bell, K. (2013). 'Prejudice', *Open Education Sociology Dictionary* [Online]. Available at: https://sociologydictionary.org/prejudice/ (Accessed: 19 July 2019).

Benner, P. (1982). 'From novice to expert', *American Journal of Nursing*, 82(3), 402–407.

Bhopal, K. and Alibhai-Brown, Y. (2018). *White Privilege: The Myth of a Post-Racial Society*. Bristol: Policy Press.

Bourdieu, P. and Passeron, J. (1990). *Reproduction in Education, Society and Culture*. 2nd edn. Thousand Oaks, CA: Sage.

Bravette, G. (1997). *Transforming Lives: Towards Bicultural Competence: Researching for Personal and Professional Transformation*. PhD dissertation. Bath: University of Bath.

Brown, R. (1995). *Prejudice: Its Social Psychology*. Oxford: Blackwell Publishers Ltd.

Burns, W. E. (2001). *The Scientific Revolution: An Encyclopedia*. Santa Barbara, CA: ABC-CLIO.

Carter, B. (2002). *Realism and Racism: Concepts of Race in Sociological Research*. Abingdon: Routledge.

Chiavaroli, N. and Trumble, S. (2018). 'When I say … phronesis', *Medical Education*, 52(10), pp.1005–1007.

Cole, E.R. and Harper, S.R. (2017). 'Race and rhetoric: An analysis of college presidents' statements on campus racial incidents', *Journal of Diversity in Higher Education*, 10(4), pp.318–333.

Cole, M. (2007). *Marxism and Educational Theory: Origins and Issues*. Abingdon-on-Thames: Taylor and Francis.

Cregan, E. (2010). *Independence and Equality (World Black History)*. Oxford: Raintree.

Crenshaw, K., Gotanda, N., Peller, G. and Thomas, K. (1996). *Critical Race Theory: The Key Writings that Formed the Movement*. New York: The New Press.

Crenshaw, K. (1988). 'Race, reform, and retrenchment: Transformation and legitimation in antidiscrimination law', *Harvard Law Review*, 101, p.1331.

Crotty, M.J. (1998). *The Foundations of Social Research: Meaning and Perspective in the Research Process*. Thousand Oaks, CA: Sage Publishing.

Delgado Bernal, D. (1998). 'Using a Chicana feminist epistemology in educational research', *Harvard Educational Review*, 68(4), pp.555–582.

Delgado-Bernal, D. (2002). 'Critical race theory, Latino critical theory and critical raced-gendered epistemologies: Recognizing Students of Color as holders and creators of knowledge', *Qualitative Inquiry*, 8(1), pp.105–126.

Denzin, N. and Lincoln, Y. (2011). *The Discipline and Practice of Qualitative Research*. London: Sage.

DiAngelo, R. (2011). 'White fragility', *International Journal of Critical Pedagogy*, 3(3), pp.54–70.

DiAngelo, R. (2018). *White Fragility*. London: Penguin Random House UK.

Douglas, F. (1995). *The Color Line*. Charlottesville, Virginia: University of Virginia.

Dovidio, J. and Gaertner, S. (2010). 'Intergroup bias' in Fiske, S.T., Gilbert, D.T. and Lindzey, G. (eds) *The Handbook of Social Psychology*. 5th edn. New York: Wiley. pp. 1084–1121

Eisner, E.W. (1991). *The Enlightened Eye: Qualitative Inquiry and the Enhancement of Educational Practice*. New York: Macmillan Publishing Company.

Employment Law Clinic. (2018). *Disciplinary Action Flowchart – Guide for a Disciplinary Process* [Online]. Available at: http://employmentlawclinic.com/disciplinary-action-flowchart/#flowchart (Accessed: 11 June 2018).

Equality and Human Rights Commission. (2019). *What Is Discrimination* [Online]. Available at: https://www.equalityhumanrights.com/en/advice-and-guidance/what-discrimination (Accessed: 9 April 2021).

Equality and Human Rights Commission. (2021). *Public Sector Equality Duty* [Online]. Available at: https://www.equalityhumanrights.com/ en/advice-and-guidance/public-sector-equality-duty (Accessed: 31 March 2021).

Equality Hub. (2016). *Age* [Online]. Available at: https://equalityhub.org/2016/07/06/age/ (Accessed: 4 January 2017).

Equal Opportunities Commission. (2021). *What Is Discrimination* [Online]. Available at: https://www.eoc.org.uk/what-is-discrimination/ (Accessed: 9 April 2021).

Federal Bureau of Investigation. (2016). *Civil Rights* [Online]. Available at: https://www.fbi.gov/investigate/civil-rights (Accessed: 9 March 2021).

Fine, M. (1997). 'Witnessing whiteness' in Fine, M., Weis, L., Powell, C. and Wong, L. (eds) *Off White: Readings on Race, Power, and Society*. Abingdon: Routledge. pp.57–65.

Fish, G. and Syed, M. (2019). *The Multiple Levels of Racism, Discrimination, and Prejudice*. Minneapolis, MN: University of Minnesota Press.

Flowers, K., Reid, P. and Larkin, P. (2005). 'Exploring lived experience'. *The Psychologist,* 18, pp.20–23.

Frankenberg, R. (1993). *White Women, Race Matters: The Social Construction of Whiteness*. Minneapolis, MN: University of Minnesota Press.

GOV.UK. (2016). *The NHS Constitution for England.* [Online] Available at: https://www.gov.uk/government/publications/the-nhs-constitution-for-england/the-nhs-constitution-for-england (Accessed: 24 July 2017).

Hall, B. (2005). *Among Cultures: The Challenge of Communication*. Belmont, CA: Thompson Wadsworth.

Hefferman, M. (2014). *How Can We Combat Wilful Blindness to Ensure a Culture of Quality?* Available at: https://www.kingsfund.org.uk/sites/default/files/media/Heffernan.pdf (Accessed: 21 June 2020).

Henry, Z. (1985). 'The New Commonwealth Migrants 1945-62', *History Today*, 35(12) [Online]. Available at: https://www.historytoday.com/archive/new-commonwealth-migrants-1945-62 (Accessed: 11 September 2015).

Hilliard, A. (1992). *Racism: Its Origins and How It Works*. Paper presented at the meeting of the Mid-West Association for the Education of Young Children. Madison, WI.

Hirsch, A. (2020). 'The 'playing the race card' accusation is just a way to silence us', *The Guardian*, 16 January [Online]. Available at: https://www.theguardian.com/commentisfree/2020/jan/16/playing-the-race-card-racism-black-experience (Accessed: 21 January 2020).

Home Office. (1999). 'The Stephen Lawrence inquiry', *GOV.UK*, 24 February [Online]. Available at: https://www.gov.uk/government/publications/the-stephen-lawrence-inquiry (Accessed: 3 November 2018).

Huber, L. (2008). 'Building critical race methodologies in educational research: A research note on critical race testimonio', *FIU Law Review*, 4(1) [Online]. Available at: https://ecollections.law.fiu.edu/cgi/viewcontent.cgi?article=1052andcontext= lawreview (Accessed: 12 June 2015).

John, G. (2014). *Global African Diaspora: Transforming the State We're In?* [Online]. Available at: https://www.obv.org.uk/news-blogs/global-african-diaspora-transforming-state-we-re (Accessed: 6 February 2019).

John, G. (2015*). Eulogy - Celebrating Jean Mary Griffiths*. 24 February, Cathedral of the Immaculate Conception, Grenada.

Jones, J. (1997). *Prejudice and Racism*. 2nd edn. New York: McGraw-Hill.

Jones, T. (2000). 'Shades of brown: The law of skin color', *Duke Law Journal*, 49(6) [Online]. Available at: doi:10.2139/ssrn.233850 (Accessed: 8 July 2019).

Jones-Berry, S. (2017). 'Racism in the NHS: are things getting better or worse for BME staff?', *Nursing Standard,* 2 October [Online]. Available at: https://rcni. com/nursing-standard/newsroom/analysis/racism-nhs-are-things-getting-better-or-worse-bme-staff-152681 (Accessed: 20 March 2020).

Keogh, K. (2019). 'NHS becoming less diverse at board level, report reveals', *Nursing Standard,* 8 June [Online]. Available at: https://rcni.com/nursing-standard/ newsroom/news/nhs-becoming-less-diverse-board-level-report-reveals-149871 (Accessed: 10 June 2019).

Kinsella, E. and Pitman, A. (2012). *Phronesis as Professional Knowledge: Practical Wisdom in the Professions*. Rotterdam: Sense Publishers.

Kivel, P. (2017). *Uprooting Racism 4th Edition – Paul Kivel*. [Online]. Available at: http://paulkivel.com/books/uprooting-racism-4th-edition/ (Accessed: 23 October 2019).

Kline, R. (2014). *The "Snowy White Peaks" of the NHS: A Survey of Discrimination in Governance and Leadership and the Potential Impact on Patient Care in London and England* [Online]. Available at: www.mdx.ac.uk/__data/.../The-snowy-white-peaks-of-the-NHS.pdf (Accessed: 7 June 2015).

Kline, R. and Prabhu, U. (2015), 'Race inequality of NHS staff is putting patients at risk', *Health Service Journal* [Online]. Available at: https://www.hsj.co.uk/ leadership/race-inequality-of-nhs-staff-is-putting-patients-at-risk/5082766.article (Accessed: 3 August 2020).

Knaus, C. (2018). 'Mehreen Faruqi warns against "normalisation" of racism in first Senate speech', *The Guardian*, 21 August [Online]. Available at: https://www. theguardian.com/australia-news/2018/aug/21/mehreen-faruqi-warns-against-normalisation-of-racism-in-first-senate-speech (Accessed: 25 March 2020).

Kolb, D.A. (1984). *Experiential Learning: Experience as the Source of Learning and Development*. Englewood Cliffs, NJ: Prentice-Hall.

Ladson-Billings, G. and Tate, W.F. (2000). 'From the editors', *American Educational Research Journal*, 37(1), pp.305–305.

Lais, H. (2019). 'Racism is rife in modern Britain. Nothing can change until we admit it'. *The Independent*, 25 October [Online]. Available at: https://www.independent. co.uk/voices/black-history-month-racism-institutional-britain-slavery-education-employment-culture-colonialism-a9170841.html (Accessed: 25 June 2020).

Lamuye, A. (2017). 'I am no "person of colour", I am a black African woman,' Independent, 31 July [Online]. Available at: https://www.independent.co.uk/voices/ phrase-people-person-of-colour-bme-black-woman-women-different-experiences-race-racism-a7868586.html (Accessed 16 June 2020).

Laverack, G. (2005). *Public Health, Power, Empowerment and Professional Practice*. Basingstoke: Palgrave Macmillan.

Lee Hall, R. (2016). *Denying Racism Is the New Racism* [Online]. Available at: https://ezinearticles.com/?Denying-Racism-Is-the-New-Racismandid=9562754 (Accessed: 4 January 2020).

Letts, L. (2003). 'Occupational therapy and participatory research: A partnership worth pursuing', *American Journal of Occupational Therapy*, 57, pp.77–87.

Letts, L., Wilkins, S., Law, M., Stewart, D., Bosch, J., & Westmorland, M. (2007). *Critical Review Form – Qualitative Studies* (Version 2.0). McMaster University.

LinkedIn. (2015). *Core Values – Why Are They so Important to Your Company?* [Online]. Available at: https://www.linkedin.com/pulse/core-values-why-so-important-your-company-nicolas-schoenlaub/ (Accessed: 3 August 2020).

López, G.R. (2001). 'Re-Visiting White Racism in Educational Research: Critical Race Theory and the Problem of Method', *Educational Researcher*, 30(1), pp.29–33.

Marshall, C. and Rossman, G. (2006). *Designing Qualitative Research*. 4th edn. Thousands Oaks, CA: Sage Publication.

McCalla, C. (2011). 'The top 5 assassinations of black leaders,' *Newsone*, 26 October [Online]. Available at: https://newsone.com/1602245/top-5-assassinations-black-leaders (Accessed: 26 March 2020).

Mcintosh, P. (1989). *White Privilege: Unpacking the Invisible Knapsack*. [Online]. Available at: https://psychology.umbc.edu/files/2016/10/White-Privilege_McIntosh-1989.pdf (Accessed: 20 November 2019).

Mehra, B. (2002). 'Bias in qualitative research: voices from an online classroom,' *The Qualitative Report*, 7(1), pp.1–19.

Merrifield, N. (2015). 'Nursing debate questions long-term impact of "6Cs" values', *Nursing Times* [Online]. Available at: https://www.nursingtimes.net/archive/nursing-debate-questions-long-term-impact-of-6cs-values-23-03-2015/ (Accessed: 20 March 2019).

Moustakas, C. (1994). *Phenomenological Research Methods*. Thousand Oaks, CA: Sage.

Nadeem, S. (2019). *Evaluation of the NHS Workforce Race Equality Standard (WRES)*. [Online]. Available at: https://www.england.nhs.uk/wp-content/uploads/2019/09/wres-evaluation-report-january-2019.pdf (Accessed: 21 November 2019).

Naylor, D. (2008). *An Investigation Into How Public Sector and Community-Based Practitioners Authorise Constructively Awkward Interventions* [Online]. Available at: http://eprints.mdx.ac.uk/6894/ (Accessed: 16 April 2017).

NHS Digital. (2022). *NHS Vacancy Statistics England April 2015 – December 2021 Experimental Statistics*. [Online]. Available at: https://digital.nhs.uk/ data-and-information/publications/statistical/nhs-vacancies-survey/april-2015 – december-2021-experimental-statistics# (Accessed: 4 October 2022).

NHS England. (2016). *Workplace Experiences of BME and White Staff Published for Every NHS Trust Across England*. [Online]. Available at: https://www.england.nhs.uk/2016/06/wres-publication/ (Accessed: 16 June 2020).

NHS WRES. (2019). *2018 Data Analysis Report for NHS Trusts* [Online]. Available at: https://www.england.nhs.uk/wp-content/uploads/2018/12/wres-2018-report-v1.pdf (Accessed: 20 August 2019).

NMC.Org. UK. (2017). *The NMC Register.* [Online]. Available at: https://www.nmc.org.uk/globalassets/sitedocuments/data-reports/the-nmc-register-30-september-2017.pdf (Accessed: 3rd October 2019).

Ortlipp, M. (2008). 'Keeping and using reflective journals in the qualitative research process', *The Qualitative Report, 13*(4), pp.695–705.

Owuor, M. (2017). *What Is Systemic Racism?* [Online]. Available at: worldatlas.com/articles/what-is-systemic-racism.html (Accessed: 5 August 2020).

Smith, J. and Osborn, M. (2015). 'Interpretative phenomenological analysis as a useful methodology for research on the lived experience of pain,' *British Journal of Pain, 9*(1), pp.41–42.

Sofaer, S. (1999). *Qualitative Methods: What Are They and Why Use Them?* [Online]. Available at: http://www.ncbi.nlm.nih.gov/pubmed/10591275 (Accessed: 20 March 2014).

Sue, D.W. (2010). *Micro-aggressions in Everyday Life: Race, Gender and Sexual Orientation.* 1st edn. New York: Wiley.

Sultana, F. (2007). 'Reflexivity, positionality and participatory ethics: Negotiating fieldwork dilemmas in international research', *ACME, 6*(3), pp.374–385.

Tahan, H.A. and Sminkey, P. (2012). 'Motivational interviewing: building rapport with clients to encourage desirable behavioural and lifestyle changes', *Professional Case Management, 17*(4), pp.164–172.

TB Facts. (2018). *TB Facts – Information about TB – TB Facts* [Online]. Available at: https://tbfacts.org/ (Accessed: 5 May 2019).

The Institute of Race Relations. (2017). *Definitions* [Online]. Available at: http://www.irr.org.uk/research/statistics/definitions/ (Accessed: 5 July 2017).

The Royal College of Nursing. (2018). *RCN Bulletin 368: October 2018* [Online]. Available at: https://www.rcn.org.uk/news-and-events/rcn-magazines/bul-368 (Accessed: 3 October 2019).

The Royal College of Nursing. (2019). *Rise in reported racial discrimination in the NHS a disgrace* [Online]. Available at: https://www.rcn.org.uk/news-and-events/news/rise-in-reported-racial-discrimination-in-the-nhs-a-disgrace. (Accessed: 3 April 2019).

Utley, E.A. (2016). 'Humanizing Blackness: An Interview with Tommy J. Curry,' *Southern Communication Journal, 81*(4), pp.263–266.

Vonderbeck, R. and Worth, N. (2015). *Intergenerational Space.* London: Routledge

Watson-Druee, N. (2009). 'Why BME nurses lack opportunities in today's NHS', *Nursing Times,* 20 April [Online]. Available at: https://www.nursingtimes.net/why-bme-nurses-lack-opportunities-in-todays-nhs/5000641.article (Accessed: 2 April 2017).

Wilson, J. (2018). 'NHS increasingly desperate for nurses and midwives as applications continue to fall,' *The Telegraph,* 27 July [Online]. Available at: https://www.telegraph.co.uk/news/2018/07/27/nhs-increasingly-desperate-nurses-midwives-applications-continue/ (Accessed: 24 January 2020).

Worchel, S., Rothgerber, H., Day, E.A., Hart, D. and Butemeyer, J. (1998). 'Social identity and individual productivity within groups,' *British Journal of Social Psychology, 37*(4), pp.389–413.

Yosso, T.J. (2005). 'Whose culture has capital? A critical race theory discussion of community cultural wealth,' *Race Ethnicity and Education, 8*(1), pp.69–91.

Index

For Product Safety Concerns and Information please contact our EU
representative GPSR@taylorandfrancis.com
Taylor & Francis Verlag GmbH, Kaufingerstraße 24, 80331 München, Germany

www.ingramcontent.com/pod-product-compliance
Lightning Source LLC
Chambersburg PA
CBHW060312220326
41598CB00027B/4311